STECK-VAUGHN

Decisions for Health

THE COMPLETE EDITION

VIVIAN BERNSTEIN

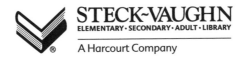

STECK-VAUGHN
ELEMENTARY · SECONDARY · ADULT · LIBRARY

A Harcourt Company

www.steck-vaughn.com

About the Author

Vivian Bernstein has been a teacher in the New York City Public School System for a number of years. She received her Master of Arts degree from New York University. Bernstein is active with professional organizations in social studies, education, and reading. She gives presentations to school faculties and professional groups about content area reading. Bernstein is the author of *America's Story, World History and You, World Geography and You,* and *American Government.*

Acknowledgments

Cover: Cooke Photographics; p.3 © Bob Daemmrich/Stock Boston; pp.4–5 © Bob Daemmrich/Stock Boston; p.6 © Richard Hutchings/Photo Researchers; p.7 © David Young Wolff/PhotoEdit; p.11 © L. Druskis/Photo Researchers; p.12 © Michael Grecco/Stock Boston; p.13 © Tony Freeman/PhotoEdit; p.14 © Bob Kramer/Stock Boston; p.15 © MacDonald Photography/Unicorn Stock; p.16 © Michael Dwyer/Stock Boston; p.17 © Steve Bourgeois/Unicorn Stock; p.20 © Mary Kate Denny/PhotoEdit; p.21 © Stephen McBrady/PhotoEdit; p.22 © Richard Hutchings/PhotoEdit; p.23 James Minor; p.24 © Richard Hutchings/PhotoEdit; p.27 © Tony Freeman/PhotoEdit; p.28 © Bob Daemmrich/Stock Boston; p.29 © Tony Freeman/PhotoEdit; p.30 © Richard Hutchings/Photo Researchers; p.31 © Richard Hutchings/PhotoEdit; p.35 © Bob Daemmrich/Stock Boston; p.36 © Robert Brenner/PhotoEdit; p.37 © Tony Freeman/PhotoEdit; p.40 © Jeffry Myers/Stock Boston; p.51 © Bryce Flynn/Stock Boston; p.52 © Myrleen Ferguson/PhotoEdit; p.53 Susan Rosenberg/Photo Researchers; p.57 © Chris Brown/Unicorn Stock Photos; p.58 © Tony Freeman/PhotoEdit; p.59 © Tony Freeman/PhotoEdit; p.60 © George Bellerose/Stock Boston; p.61 (all) © Park Street; p.64 © Stephen Frisch/Stock Boston; p.66 ©Tom Prettyman/PhotoEdit; p.67 © Bob Daemmrich/Stock Boston; p.70 © Sylvia Miller/Custom Medical Stock; p.71 © Edward H. Gill/Custom Medical Stock; p.72 © Barbara Alper/Stock Boston; p.73 (both) © Judy Gelles/Stock Boston; p.76 © Michael Hayman/Stock Boston; p.77 © Park Street; p.78 © Tony Freeman/PhotoEdit; p.79 © David M. Grossman/Photo Researchers; p.82 © Richard Hutchings/PhotoEdit; p.83 © Gary Weber/Photo Researchers; p.84 © Park Street; p.85 © Bob Daemmrich/Stock Boston.; p.89 © Miro Vintoniv/Stock Boston; p.90 © Frances Cox/Stock Boston; p.91 © Robert Brenner/PhotoEdit; p.92 © Richard Hutchings/PhotoEdit; p.93 © Mary Kate Denny/PhotoEdit; p.94 © Tony Freeman/PhotoEdit; p.97 © Tony Freeman/PhotoEdit; p.98 © Barbara Rios/Photo Researchers; p.99 © Rich Baker/Unicorn Stock Photos; p.100 © Charles E. Schmidt/Unicorn Stock Photos; p.101 © Ulrike Welsch/Photo Researchers; p.102 © Jean-Claude Lejeune/Stock Boston; p.105 © Blair Seitz/Photo Researchers; p.106 © Mary Kate Denny/PhotoEdit; p.107 James Minor; p.108 © Robert Pearcy/Animals, Animals; p.109 © Owen Franken/Stock Boston; p.110 © Seth Resnick/Stock Boston; p.111 © Richard Hutchings/PhotoEdit; p.114 © Peter Menzel/Stock Boston; p.116 © Fritz Henle/Photo Researchers (hurricane); p.116 © D. Bretzfelder/PhotoEdit; p.117 © Barbara Alper/Stock Boston.; p.121 © Blair Seitz/Photo Researchers; p.122 © Park Street; p.123 © Ken Lax/Photo Researchers; p.124 © Joseph Nettis/Photo Researchers; p.125 © Michael Newman/PhotoEdit; p.126 © Richard Hutchings/Photo Researchers; p.130 © Park Street; p.131 © Park Street; p.132 American Arthritis Foundation; p.134 AP/Wide World; p.137 © Michael Newman/PhotoEdit; p.138 © Bohdan Mrynewych/Stock Boston; p.139 © Kathy Sloane/Photo Researchers; p. 140 © Rhoda Sidney/PhotoEdit. Continued on page 313.

Consultants:

Lori A. Hagen: Ms. Hagen is a special education teacher in Albuquerque, New Mexico.

Elnora P. Mendías, MS, RN, CFNP: Ms. Mendías is a doctoral candidate at The University of Texas at Austin School of Nursing.

Credits:

Executive Editor: Diane Sharpe
Senior Editor: Martin S. Saiewitz
Project Editor: Meredith Edgley
Design Manager: Richard Balsam
Designer: John J. Harrison
Photo Editor: Margie Foster
Production: Tracor Publications
Illustrations: Accurate Art, Inc.; John J. Harrison

ISBN 0-8114-7788-6

CONTENTS

CONTENTS

CONTENTS

CONTENTS

To the Reader

What are some of the things you want? You may want new shoes, nice clothes, or a new bike. But one of the most important things you should want is good health. Having good health will help you enjoy life.

There are many ways you can improve your health. You can exercise to make your body stronger. You can learn how to be safe when you are at home and away from home. You can learn to choose products and services that are good for your health.

To be healthy you must make many kinds of decisions. Your decisions should help you choose healthy foods, activities, and behaviors. Good health habits help you avoid disease. You can protect your body with a diet that is low in fat. You can build a strong heart by exercising at least three times a week. Getting along with your family and friends is another way you can protect your health.

To be healthy you must avoid behaviors that can be harmful. Smoking cigarettes damages your heart and lungs. Alcohol and drug abuse can destroy your health. You can also harm yourself with risk behaviors or poor health habits that lead to diseases.

As you read *Decisions for Health*, you will learn how to improve your health. You will learn how to handle your feelings, solve problems, and set goals. You will also learn how to care for your body, protect it, and keep it strong. You will learn how to avoid harmful behaviors.

The health skills you learn in this book will help you every day of the year. Making good health habits part of your life will help you enjoy many years of good health.

UNIT 1

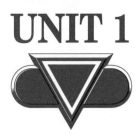

Wellness

Have you ever watched the Olympics on TV? If you did, you saw some of the world's best runners, swimmers, and skaters. These people in the Olympics had goals. Their goals were to win the Olympic medals. To reach their goals, they needed good health. Good health helped them become winners.

Most of us will never be in the Olympics. But we have other goals we want to reach. Having good health helps us reach our goals.

Have You Ever Wondered?

▼ Being healthy means more than being strong and athletic. What can you do to be healthy?

▼ Your highest health goal should be wellness. What is wellness?

▼ The way you get along with people affects your health. Why do some people make friends easily?

▼ Making wise decisions helps you have good health. How can you make wise decisions?

As you read this unit, think about the ways good health can make your life better.

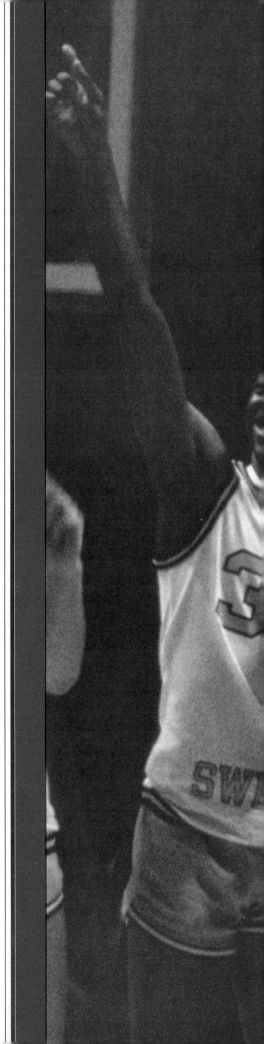

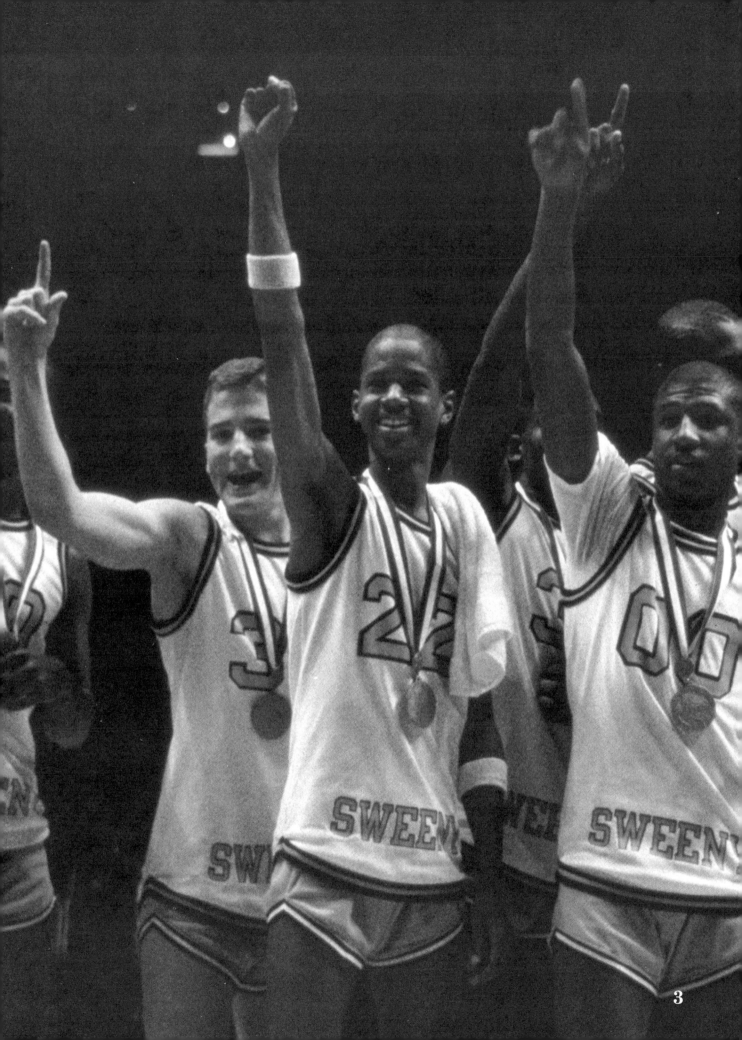

Choosing Good Health

Think About as You Read

- Why should wellness be your health goal?
- How can risk behaviors hurt your health?
- How can wise decision making help you have good health?

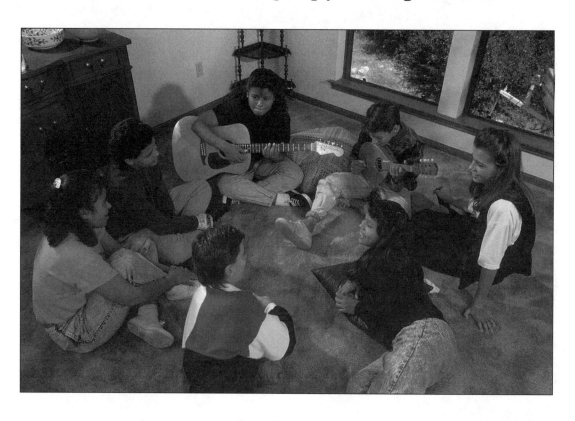

Good health allows you to enjoy life.

Imagine you are at a party. There is a lot of good food and music. You want to have a good time. Can you enjoy yourself if you start to feel sick? Will you have fun if you don't get along with the people at the party? Can you have a good time if you have sad and angry feelings? Having good health will help you enjoy the party. Good health allows you to enjoy your life. As you read this book, you will learn how to care for your health.

What Is Wellness?

Many people have health goals. The highest health goal is **wellness**. Wellness means more than not being sick. Wellness means having good physical, social, and emotional health.

Physical health is how you take care of your body. Eating healthy foods helps you have good physical health. You take care of your physical health when you get enough sleep and exercise.

Social health is the way you get along with others. Good social health means you try to get along with your family and friends. You care about and help others.

Emotional health is the way you live with your feelings. Good emotional health means that you have good feelings about yourself. Knowing how to make wise decisions helps you have good emotional health.

Risk Behaviors Can Hurt Your Health

People who want to reach the goal of wellness avoid **risk behaviors**. Smoking cigarettes and eating too much food are risk behaviors that harm your physical health. Risk behaviors stop people from reaching the goal of wellness.

All **risk behaviors** are actions that can harm your physical, social, or emotional health.

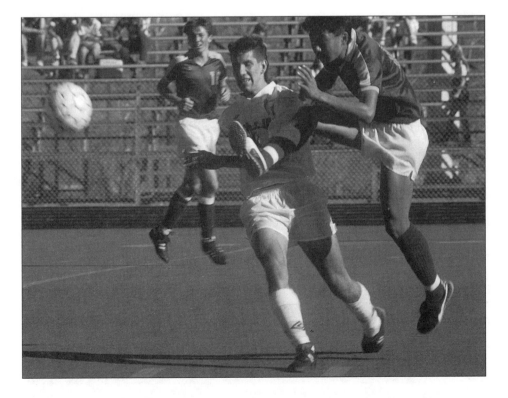

Playing sports can help you improve your physical, social, and emotional health.

To reach the goal of wellness, people make decisions to avoid risk behaviors. One decision might be to wear a seat belt when riding in a car. Seat belts help protect you in car accidents. Another decision for wellness might be to eat fewer foods with sugar. You protect your teeth by eating less sugar.

Decision Making and Wellness

You make many decisions each day. Wise decision making helps you reach wellness. Some decisions are simple. A simple decision might be whether to eat a plain baked potato or French fries for dinner. Since French fries are cooked in oil, they are the less healthy food. The healthier choice is the plain baked potato. Other decisions are more difficult. It is harder to decide how to use your time after school. Should you get a job or join a club? Should you spend more time studying?

Learning to make wise decisions is important. You can use these six steps to help you make decisions.

1. Understand the problem. You must feel that a decision is needed.
2. Think about two or three choices that can solve the problem.

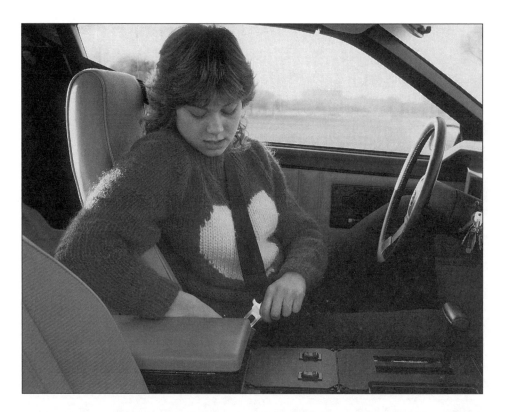

Wearing seat belts protects you from being hurt during car accidents.

6

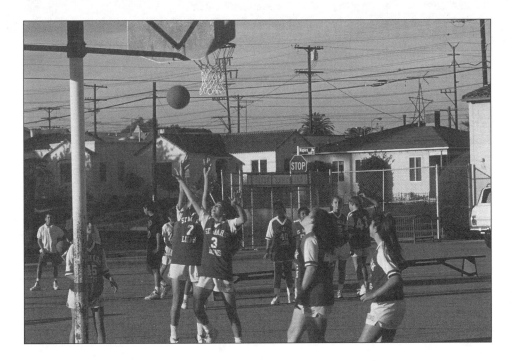

Joining a sports team can help you have fun, make friends, and improve your skills.

3. Think about the possible **consequence** of each choice.
4. Pick the choice that you think is best.
5. Put your decision into action.
6. Think about your decision. Would you use this decision to solve this problem again?

A **consequence** is the result of a decision or action.

Let's put the decision-making steps to work. Jessica wanted to be on the school basketball team. The team played every Wednesday afternoon. She was also offered a baby-sitting job near her house. The job was for three afternoons a week. Jessica had to decide whether to join the basketball team or to accept the job. She thought about both choices. If she joined the basketball team, she would enjoy being with friends. She would also improve her basketball skills. If she took the job, she would earn money to spend on extra things she wanted. But Jessica also knew she would have less time for fun or for studying three afternoons each week. Jessica decided to join the basketball team. After she had a great time at the first game, she knew she had made the right decision.

As you read this book, you will learn how to work toward the goal of wellness. Good health will help you enjoy your life today and every day.

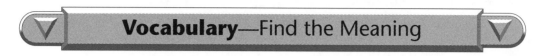

Using What You Learned

Vocabulary—Find the Meaning

Number your paper from 1 to 5. Write on your paper the word or words that best complete each sentence.

1. Eating healthy foods and getting enough sleep and exercise help you have good _____ .

   social health   **health goals**   **physical health**

2. You can reach your goal of wellness if you avoid _____ .

   decision making   **risk behaviors**   **healthy foods**

3. The way you get along with others is your _____ .

   social health   **consequence**   **risk behaviors**

4. Every decision you make has a _____ .

   winner   **social health**   **consequence**

5. _____ means having good physical, social, and emotional health.

   Consequences   **Wellness**   **Risk behaviors**

Comprehension—Write the Answer

Number your paper from 1 to 5. Write a sentence on your paper to answer each question.

1. Why is wellness an important health goal?

2. What can you do to take care of your physical health?

3. Why should you avoid risk behaviors?

4. Why is making wise decisions important?

5. What is the first step in making a wise decision?

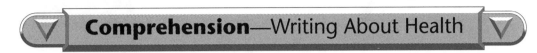
Answer the following question in complete sentences on your paper.

What decisions have you made today that will help you reach the goal of wellness?

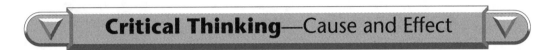

Critical Thinking—Cause and Effect

A **cause** is something that makes something else happen. What happens is called the **effect**.

> **Cause**   You start to feel sick at a party,
>
> **Effect**   so you leave the party.

Number your paper from 1 to 6. Write sentences on your paper by matching each cause on the left with an effect on the right.

Cause

1. Wellness is your highest health goal, so _____

2. The skater's physical health is important to her, so _____

3. You make several decisions every day, so _____

4. You are eating too much, so _____

5. Lisa smokes cigarettes, so _____

6. You want to be safe in your car, so _____

Effect

a. she gets plenty of sleep and exercise.

b. she is harming her physical health.

c. you wear your seat belt.

d. you learn how to make wise decisions.

e. you work toward having good physical, social, and emotional health.

f. you gain weight.

9

UNIT 2

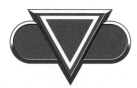

Emotional Health

Look at yourself in the mirror. Does your face show what you are feeling? Sometimes your face does show that you are feeling happy, sad, or angry. But often you are the only person who knows what kind of feelings are inside of you. To have good emotional health, you must find healthy ways to live with your feelings.

How can you have good emotional health? You need to feel good about yourself. You need goals that you can reach. You must also learn to say no when friends ask you to take part in risk behaviors. To reach your health goal of wellness, you must have good emotional health.

Have You Ever Wondered ?

▼ Your feelings affect your physical health. How does having a fight with a friend hurt your physical health?
▼ Your goals can change the way you feel about yourself. How can you reach your goals?
▼ Stress can help you or harm you. How does stress help you?

As you read this unit, think about the many ways good emotional health can help you have wellness.

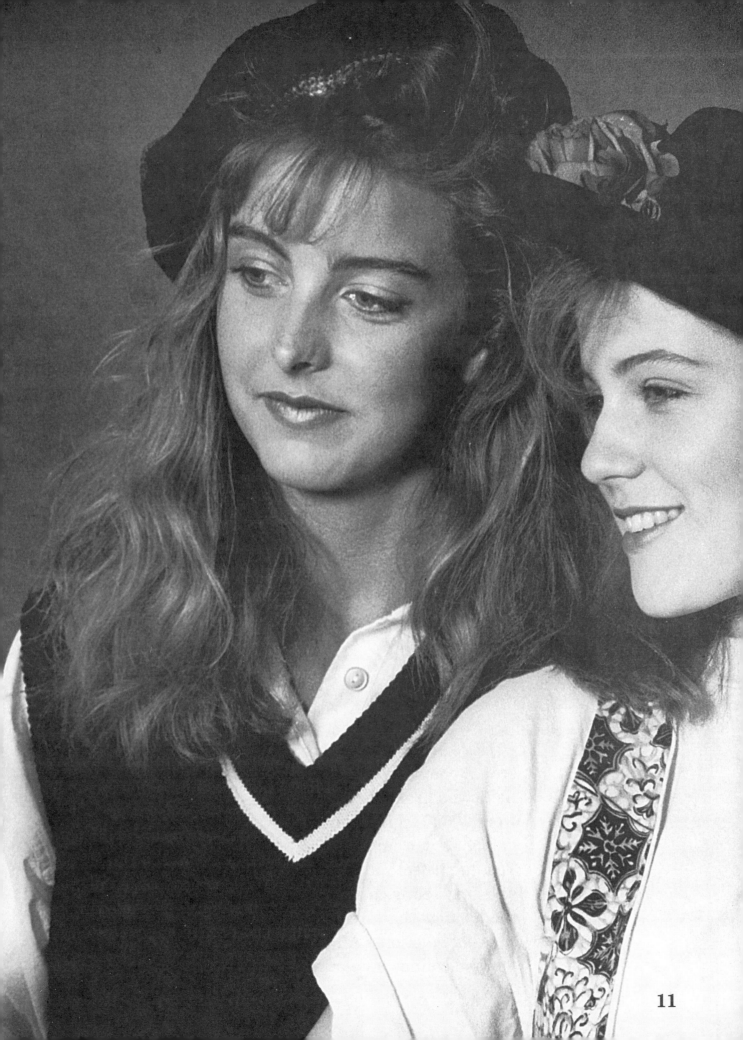

Living with Your Feelings

Think About as You Read

- **How can your feelings affect your health?**
- **What emotional needs do all people have?**
- **What happens when emotional needs are not met?**

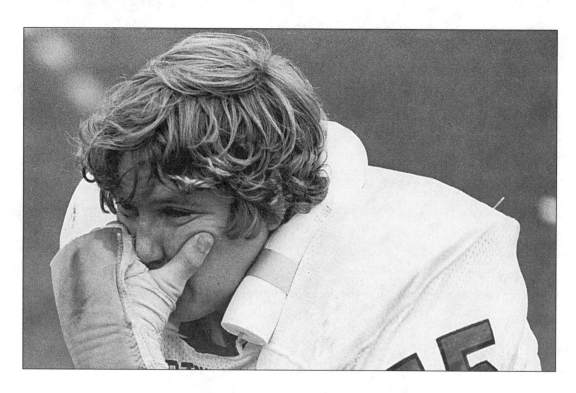

All people have emotions. What emotions do you think this football player has?

Have you ever won a prize in school? Have you ever scored points for your team during a ball game? If you have, you probably felt happy and proud. But how would you feel if you missed the ball during a ball game? How would you feel if your team lost the game? You might feel sad or angry. These happy, proud, angry, and sad feelings are called **emotions**. Emotions are the feelings that are inside of you. There are many kinds of emotions. All people have them. Emotions can also be feelings of fear, hate, and love.

The way you live with your emotions is called emotional health. Your emotional health affects the health of your body.

Emotional Health and Wellness

How does good emotional health help you have wellness? People with good emotional health care about their physical health and their social health.

People who care about their physical health take care of their bodies. They eat healthy foods and exercise. They take care of their appearance.

People with good emotional health care about their social health. They try to get along with parents, teachers, and **peers**.

Your **peers** are people who are about the same age as you.

All people sometimes feel angry, sad, and afraid. These are unpleasant emotions. You may feel better when you talk about your unpleasant feelings and problems with someone you trust. The person you talk to can be a family member, teacher, or good friend. Talking about your feelings helps your emotional health.

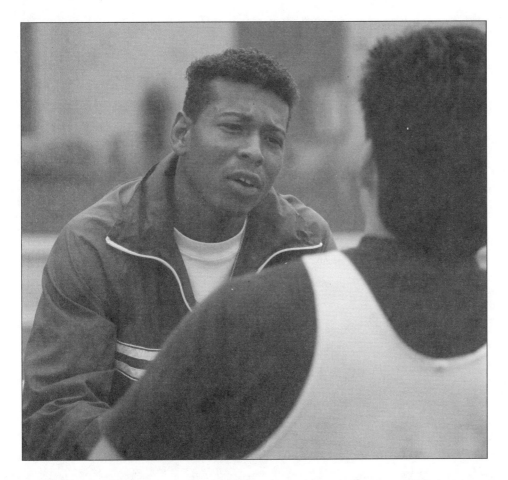

Talking to someone you trust about your unpleasant feelings helps your emotional health.

You can have poor emotional health when you feel angry, sad, or afraid most of the time. These unpleasant emotions can make you feel sick. At times they cause headaches. They can make your stomach hurt. Sometimes unpleasant feelings make it hard for you to get along with others.

Your emotions affect your emotional, physical, and social health. Have you ever had a fight with a best friend? Did that fight make you feel angry or lonely? You might have felt so unhappy about the fight that it was hard for you to eat or sleep. Or you might have said mean things to other people. Your feelings about the fight could harm your health.

Emotional Needs

All people have emotional needs. Four of the most important needs are **affection**, **acceptance**, safety, and success.

First, people need affection. They need to have good friends. They need affection from the families that they live with.

Affection is the love that you give or get from others.

Acceptance is the feeling that others like you and enjoy being with you.

Families can help each other meet their important emotional needs.

14

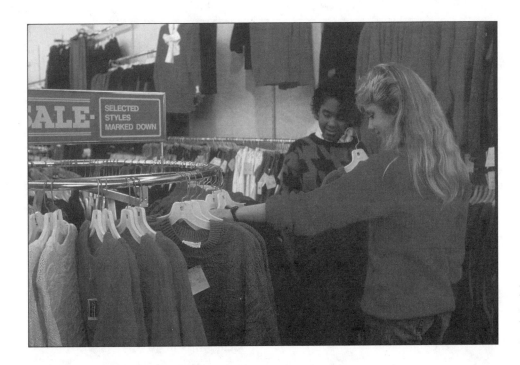

Many teen-agers feel accepted when they wear the same kind of clothes as their friends.

Second, people need acceptance. Acceptance by others is important. But people must also accept themselves. They need to feel good about themselves.

Third, people need to feel safe. They need to feel that they are not in danger.

The fourth need is success. Having good friends and making good grades in school can make a person feel successful. People feel successful when they set and reach their goals.

People use different kinds of behavior to meet their needs. To get affection from friends, a person might be helpful and friendly. To win acceptance by other teens, many teen-agers like to wear the same kind of clothes and shoes. To feel safe many bike riders wear helmets to protect their heads. Many people feel successful when they earn their own money to buy something special for themselves.

Risk Behaviors

Sometimes the four emotional needs are not met. Then angry, unhappy feelings can affect behavior and wellness. People with poor emotional health may use risk behaviors to meet their emotional needs. A person who has a fight with a best friend no longer feels the

15

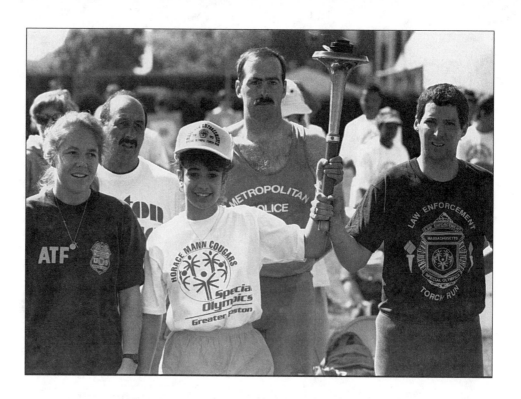

Group activities can help people meet their needs for acceptance and success.

friend's affection. That person might be angry enough to start a fight with a family member at home. Sometimes people are not accepted by their peers, so they show off to get attention.

Some people feel that they are not safe when they are away from home. So they spend as much time as they can inside their own homes. Other people feel they are not successful if they miss the ball during a ball game. Some people feel so unhappy when they miss the ball that they quit during the game. Many people choose unhealthy kinds of behavior when their emotional needs are not met.

Let's look at the risk behaviors Michael used when his needs for affection and acceptance were not met. Michael did not have friends at school. Because he felt people didn't like him, he stayed by himself most of the time. Sometimes Michael lied to his family about all the friends he had at school.

Michael should use healthy behaviors to meet his emotional needs. He could try to become friendly with one or two boys. He could also join a club or sports team. Joining a club or team could help Michael win acceptance by a group.

Good Emotional Health and Behavior

Most people have good emotional health when their emotional needs are met. If you have good emotional health, you are able to deal with problems. You can make decisions. You know you are responsible for your decisions and behavior. You can accept changes at school and at home. When you have good emotional health, you set goals for the future. You care about others and know the difference between right and wrong.

People with good emotional health **communicate** their ideas and feelings with others. Communication skills help you get along with others. Being a good listener is important for communication.

Emotional health can change and improve. It improves as you use healthy behavior to meet your emotional needs. It improves when you accept changes in your life and share your ideas and feelings with others. Good emotional health will help you reach the goal of wellness.

To **communicate** means to share your thoughts or feelings with others.

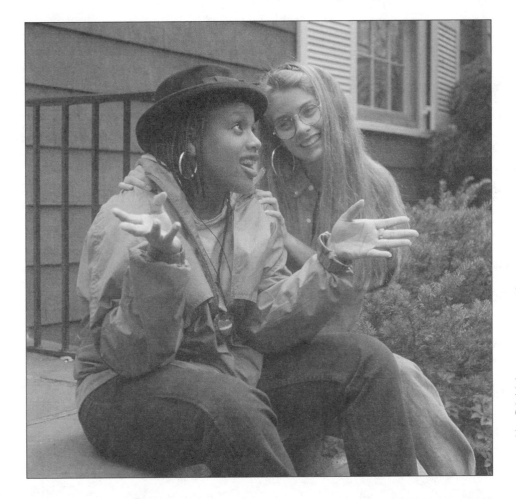

People with good emotional health care about others. They communicate their feelings.

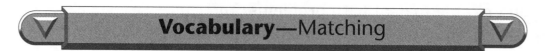

Vocabulary—Matching

Number your paper from 1 to 5. Match each vocabulary word in **Group B** with a sentence from **Group A** that tells about the word. Write the letter of the correct answer on your paper.

Group A

1. This is a person who is about your age.

2. This is the love you get from your friends and family.

3. This means to share your ideas and feelings.

4. These feelings, such as love, fear, and anger, are inside you.

5. You have this feeling when people like you and want to be with you.

Group B

a. affection

b. acceptance

c. emotions

d. communicate

e. peer

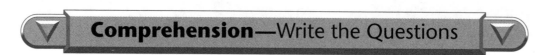

Comprehension—Write the Questions

Number your paper from 1 to 6. Below are the answers for some questions from this chapter. Read each answer. Then write on your paper a possible question to go with each answer. Use the question words to help you. The first one is done for you.

1. What **are the four most important emotional needs**?

   The four most important emotional needs are affection, acceptance, safety, and success.

2. How _____ ?

   Communication skills help you get along with others.

3. What _____ ?

Unpleasant emotions can make you feel sick.

4. Who _____ ?

A good friend will listen to you talk about your feelings.

5. What _____ ?

People with good emotional health also care about their physical health and their social health.

6. When _____ ?

People feel successful when they set and reach their goals.

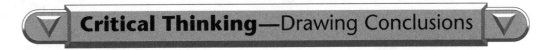

Critical Thinking—Drawing Conclusions

Read the paragraph. Then use the six steps to decide what to do about feelings of anger. Write complete sentences on your paper to answer each question.

Imagine that you have been working on a science project with your best friend. Then one day you and your friend have an argument. The argument leaves you and your friend with angry feelings toward each other. You feel like never speaking to your friend again. The next day you are still angry, but you know you need to work on the project with that friend.

Step 1. What is the problem?

Step 2. What are two ways to solve the problem?

Step 3. What is one consequence for each choice listed in Step 2?

Step 4. Which choice do you think is best?

Step 5. What can you do to put your decision into action?

Step 6. Think about your decision. Why was this the best choice for you?

Chapter 3

Feeling Good About Yourself

Think About as You Read

- How does high self-esteem help you have wellness?
- What two kinds of goals are important for self-esteem?
- How can prejudice hurt self-esteem?

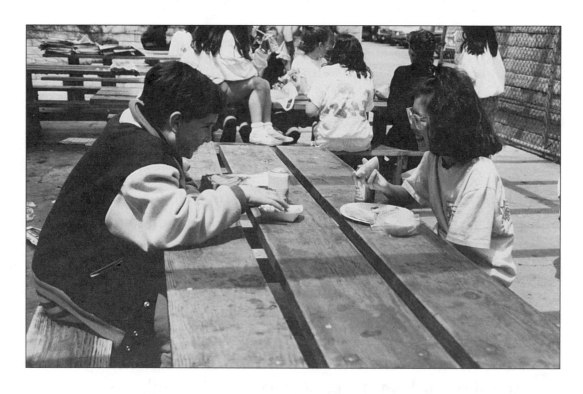

People who feel good about themselves find it easier to make friends.

During the summer Brian and his family moved to a new town. On the first day of school, Brian did not know anyone. But he remembered all the good friends he had made in his old school. He thought about how well he liked playing the drums in the band at his other school. He believed he would soon make new friends. He was sure he could join the band at the new school.

Brian has high **self-esteem**. His good feelings about himself will help him do well in his new school.

Self-Esteem, Emotional Health, and Wellness

Self-esteem is the good way you feel about yourself. You have high self-esteem if you have good feelings about yourself most of the time. You believe you can do many things well. You have low self-esteem if you do not have enough good feelings about yourself.

High self-esteem helps you have good emotional health. Your good feelings about yourself help you meet your emotional needs. You like yourself. You believe other people accept you and enjoy being with you. You make good decisions to help you stay safe. You feel successful when you set and reach your goals.

High self-esteem helps you reach the goal of wellness. When you have high self-esteem, you avoid risk behaviors. You do not want to copy any unhealthy behavior your friends may choose.

Some teens find it hard to have high self-esteem. They are not always comfortable with their changing bodies. Sometimes they cannot meet their needs for affection and acceptance. They also have trouble meeting their needs for safety and success.

When you have high self-esteem, you know you are not perfect. You believe all people are special in different ways. You are willing to learn new things. You know your weaknesses and work to improve them.

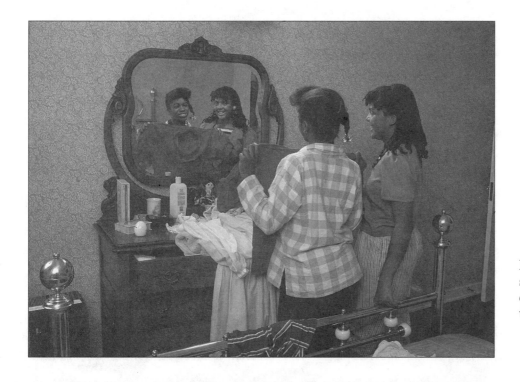

People with high self-esteem like themselves even though they know they are not perfect.

Self-Esteem and Goals

Goals are important for self-esteem. People need **long-term goals** and **short-term goals**. It may take one or more years for you to reach your long-term goals. Short-term goals can be reached in days or months. Graduating from high school is the long-term goal of many students. Your short-term goal might be to earn enough money to buy a gift for a friend.

Reaching your goals will meet your need for success. Being successful will raise your self-esteem. Try this six-step plan to reach your goals.

1. Choose goals that can be reached. Don't choose impossible goals.
2. Make a plan for reaching your goal.
3. List what you must do to reach your goal. Think about the skills you must work on.
4. Allow time to work on the goal.
5. Act on your plan.
6. Think about your goal again. Is this goal right for you? Is your plan helping you reach that goal? You might want to change your plan or your goal.

Alicia used the six-step plan to reach her goal. Her goal was to join the school chorus. Alicia asked the music teacher for the songs she would have to sing. Alicia decided to practice for 15 minutes each day.

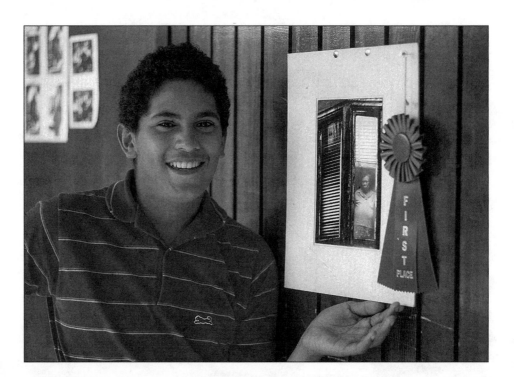

This teen's goal was to win a contest. Reaching his goal helped raise his self-esteem.

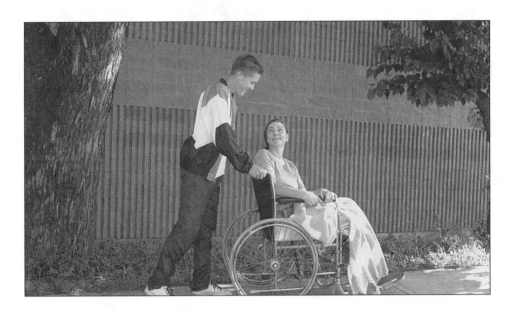

All people are special. Avoid
prejudice towards others.

She acted on her plan by singing the songs at home
each day. She tried out for the chorus, and the music
teacher asked her to join. Alicia reached her goal.
Being part of the chorus was good for her self-esteem.

Prejudice Can Hurt Self-Esteem

Some people have unfair ideas about different
groups of people. These people may think that people
who are different from them are not honest or not as
smart. These unfair ideas are **prejudices**. Some people
have prejudices about people who belong to a different
race or religion. Other people may have unfair ideas
about older adults.

Hearing other people talk about their prejudices
against you can lower your self-esteem. Imagine
hearing that the people of your race or religion are not
as smart as other people. You might hear that same
prejudice many times. After a while you might start to
believe it. You would believe you could not do as well as
other people. You might even lower your goals.

There are three kinds of behavior you can use to
avoid having prejudices. First, do not believe or say
things about people you do not know. Second, do not
make unkind jokes about people. Third, think about
how you would feel if you knew people had prejudices
against you.

Improving Your Self-Esteem

These six steps can help you raise your self-esteem.

1. Think more about the things you do well. Think less about those things you do not do as well.
2. Choose goals that you are able to reach. Choose goals for which you must do your best.
3. Accept your weak points.
4. Do your jobs for home and school.
5. Choose friends who make you feel good about yourself.
6. Join a group or a club. Work together to reach a group goal.

Ming used this six-step plan to raise his self-esteem. He knew he could draw well. He also knew he was not good at sports. So Ming joined the school art club. He made new friends who enjoyed art. Ming felt good when he saw his art club project hanging near the cafeteria. Joining the art club helped raise Ming's self-esteem.

You can raise your own self-esteem. Work at reaching your goals. Use healthy behavior to meet your emotional needs. High self-esteem will help you make responsible decisions. These decisions will help you have a healthy life.

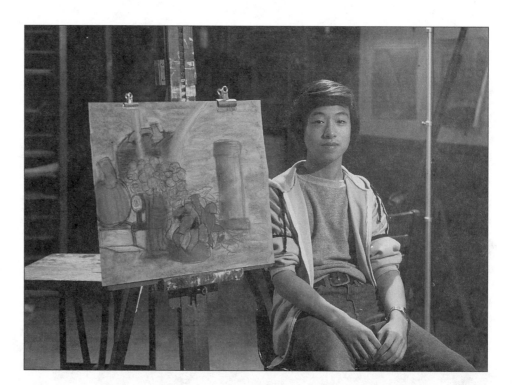

Raise your self-esteem by choosing activities that you can do well.

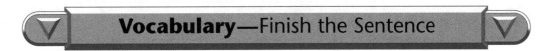

Using What You Learned

Vocabulary—Finish the Sentence

Number your paper from 1 to 6. Choose a word or words from the box to complete each sentence. Write the correct answers on your paper.

success	**short-term goal**	**self-esteem**
weaknesses	**prejudices**	**long-term goal**

1. A _____ , such as passing a math test, is a goal that can be reached quickly.

2. Feeling good about yourself and setting goals for yourself help you have high _____ .

3. Some people have _____ , which are unfair ideas about different groups of people.

4. Saving money to buy a car is a _____ because it is a goal that can take one or more years to reach.

5. Having high self-esteem means knowing your _____ and working to improve them.

6. Setting and reaching your goals will help you meet your need for _____ .

Comprehension—Writing About Health

Answer the following question in complete sentences on your paper.

What are one short-term goal and one long-term goal that you can set for yourself?

Comprehension—True or False

Write **True** on your paper for each sentence that is true. Write **False** on your paper for each sentence that is false. There are three false sentences. Rewrite the false sentences on your paper to make them true.

1. Some teens find it hard to have high self-esteem.

2. When you have high self-esteem, you know that you are perfect.

3. You want to copy your friends' unhealthy behaviors when you have high self-esteem.

4. A short-term goal might be to graduate from college.

5. Hearing other people talk about their prejudices against you can cause you to have low self-esteem.

Critical Thinking—Categories

Read the words in each group. Decide how they are alike. Find the best title in the box for each group. Write the title on your paper.

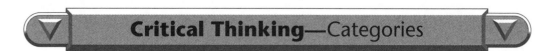

| **Short-Term Goals** | **Impossible Goals** | **High Self-Esteem** |
| **Emotional Needs** | **Long-Term Goals** | **Effects of Prejudice** |

1. finish a report
   plant a garden
   clean your room

2. like yourself
   make good decisions
   feel successful

3. get a good job
   get a driver's license
   graduate from high school

4. never make mistakes
   always be the best
   never feel angry

5. affection
   acceptance
   success

6. poor self-esteem
   lower goals
   hurt feelings

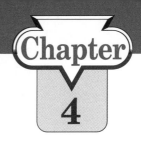

How to Live with Stress

Think About as You Read

- **How does stress affect the body?**
- **What are the causes of stress?**
- **What healthy behaviors can you use to manage stress?**

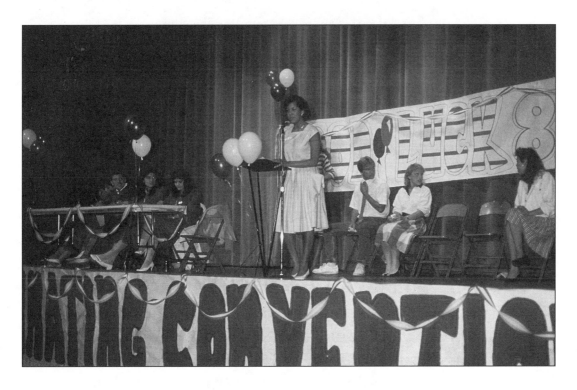

Speaking before a large group can cause stress. Stress can help you, and it can harm you.

Juan had a part in his class play. He had worked hard practicing his lines. On the day of the play, Juan felt nervous. Just before the play started, his hands began to get moist. He was afraid he would forget his lines. But when Juan went on the stage, he remembered everything. His voice was stronger than it had been all day.

Juan was suffering from **stress**. Every person feels stress each day. Sometimes stress helps us perform better. Other times we perform worse because of stress.

Stress is the way the body responds to physical, emotional, and social demands.

27

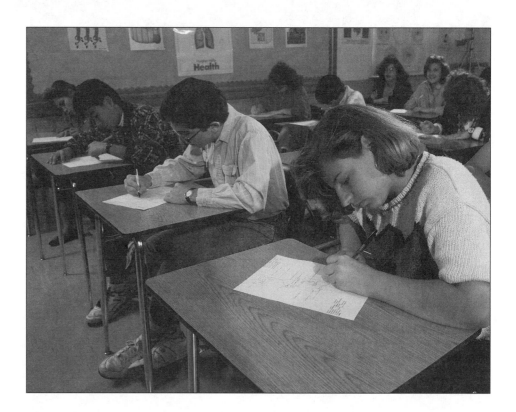

Stress might help you think better during a test.

Pressure is a strong demand.

Adrenaline is made by the body and helps prepare the body for stress.

Energy is the strength to work or do other things.

Stress and Wellness

Stress is the way the body responds to **pressure**. Physical, emotional, and social pressures cause stress. Exercise and hunger are physical pressures. Fear and anger are emotional pressures. Needing a date for a party is a social pressure.

How does the body respond to stress? It uses the **fight or flight response**. This response protects the body from stress and danger. During this response the body sends **adrenaline** into the blood. Adrenaline makes you breathe faster. It makes your heart beat faster. Adrenaline gives you extra **energy**. When the fight or flight response ends, the body returns to the way it was before the stress began.

At times stress can help you. Sometimes stress makes you feel stronger. Stress might also help you think better when you have to take a test.

Stress can also harm your body. People have more accidents when they are under stress. Stress can cause headaches. It can make your stomach and back hurt. Some people who live with a lot of stress get heart disease or other illnesses.

Stress and Your Emotional Health

Happy and sad events cause stress. A fight with a friend causes stress. Moving to a new house or having a sick parent can cause stress. Going to parties and going on dates can cause stress.

You feel stress when your emotional needs are not met. You feel stress when you do not feel loved, accepted, or successful. You also feel stress when you do not feel safe.

Unpleasant emotions, such as anger, hate, and fear, cause emotional stress. When you have these feelings often, stress can make you feel tired.

Many teen-agers feel stress because of **peer pressure**. Peer pressure might make you feel that you must wear the same shoes as your friends. You will feel stress if you want those shoes but do not have enough money to buy them.

People sometimes use risk behaviors to handle stress. They may use alcohol or drugs to feel better for a while. Other people eat too many snacks and gain weight. Risk behaviors harm your health. They never solve problems.

Peer pressure is the control over your decisions that people of your age try to have.

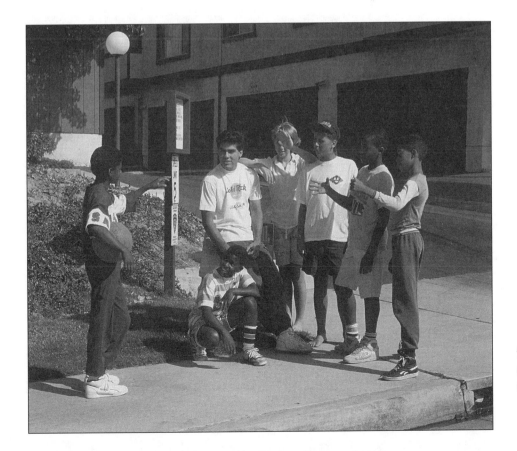

The need to be accepted and liked by your peers can cause stress.

29

Managing Stress

To reach the goal of wellness, you must use healthy behavior to help manage your stress. Here are some ways to manage stress.

1. Learn to talk about your problems and feelings. Talk to a family member, friend, or teacher that you trust. Find new ways to solve problems.
2. Find time to do something you enjoy. You may want to read or watch TV. Many people enjoy sports and music.
3. Eat healthy foods, get enough sleep, and exercise.
4. Think about the cause of your stress. Think of ways you can change whatever is causing the stress.

Say No to Peer Pressure

Peer pressure can cause you to feel a lot of stress. Deciding what to do is not always easy. Perhaps your best friend wants you to go to the movies, but you have a lot of homework. Knowing how to use the six decision-making steps from Unit 1 can help you.

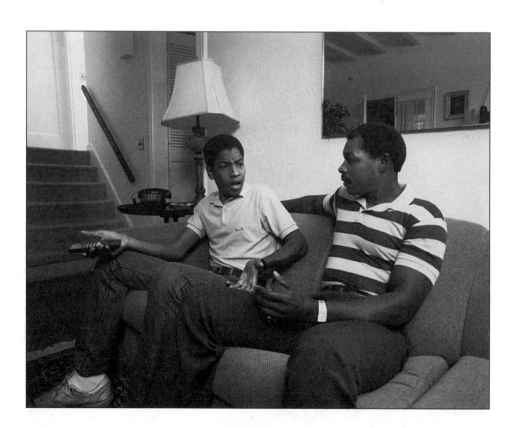

Manage your stress by talking about your feelings and problems. Talk with a person you trust.

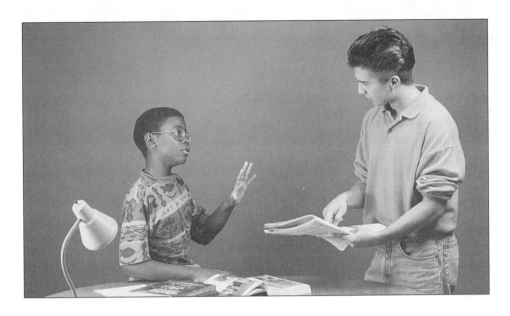

Use refusal skills to say no to peer pressure.

After you make a decision, how can you say no to peer pressure? Use **refusal skills** to say no. These four steps can help you.

1. Look at the person and say the person's name. Then say no and tell why. You might say, "Mark, I can't go to the movies. I must do my homework."
2. Ask your friend to follow your decision to choose healthy behavior. You might say, "Come over to my house. We can both do our homework."
3. Don't change your mind. You may have to repeat Step One.
4. Walk away from your friend if he or she will not accept your decision.

Karen used refusal skills to handle peer pressure. Stacey asked Karen to miss school and go shopping. Karen decided that missing school was a risk behavior. She said, "Stacey, I can't miss school. I belong in school today. I hope you'll come to school, too. We can eat lunch together." But Stacey asked Karen to go shopping again. When Karen said no, Stacey became angry. Karen walked away from her. Karen felt good about herself because she did what she thought was right. She knew she made the right decision.

Choose healthy behavior to handle stress. Use refusal skills. Good emotional health will help you reach the goal of wellness.

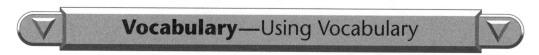

Vocabulary—Using Vocabulary

Number your paper from 1 to 6. Use the word or words to write a complete sentence on your paper about living with stress.

1. stress
2. peer pressure
3. refusal skills
4. adrenaline
5. fight or flight response
6. healthy behavior

Comprehension—Finish the Paragraph

Number your paper from 1 to 10. Use a word from the box to finish each sentence. Write the correct answers on your paper.

social	energy	decisions	perform	harmful
illnesses	behaviors	goal	cause	feels

Everyone __(1)__ stress each day. Stress is caused by physical, emotional, and __(2)__ pressures. Sometimes stress can be helpful because it makes you __(3)__ better. It can give you extra __(4)__ . But other times stress can be __(5)__ . It can __(6)__ you to have headaches. Too much stress can even cause __(7)__ , such as heart disease.

Stress can keep you from reaching your __(8)__ of wellness. You can manage stress by knowing how to make wise __(9)__ . This will help you choose healthy __(10)__ .

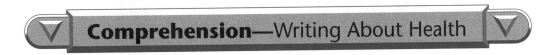

Comprehension—Writing About Health

Answer the following question in complete sentences on your paper.

What are three ways to manage stress?

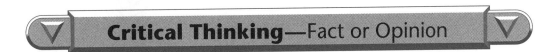

Critical Thinking—Fact or Opinion

A **fact** is a true statement. An **opinion** is a statement that tells what a person thinks.

Fact	Stress affects your body.
Opinion	It is easy to tell what causes stress.

Number your paper from 1 to 9. Write **Fact** on your paper for each fact below. Write **Opinion** for each opinion. You should find four sentences that are opinions.

1. Social pressures are not as stressful as emotional pressures.

2. The body protects itself from stress with the fight or flight response.

3. Adrenaline makes you breathe faster.

4. Happy events always cause the best kind of stress.

5. Peer pressure is a cause of stress for many teens.

6. Only athletes feel stress.

7. You might feel less stress if your emotional needs are met.

8. Reading is the best way to manage stress.

9. Anger, hate, and fear are unpleasant emotions that can cause emotional stress.

UNIT 3

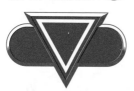

Nutrition

Think about all the food you ate yesterday. Did you eat lots of candy and fried foods? Did you eat snacks while watching TV? Were fruits and vegetables part of your meals? Perhaps you ate too much food. Or perhaps you did not eat enough food to get all the energy you need. You must make decisions about food each day. You decide what, when, and how much to eat. To reach the goal of wellness, you must learn how to make wise decisions about food.

Eating healthy foods can help us look and feel our best. Different foods help our bodies in different ways. Some foods build strong bones. Other foods give the body lots of energy. By studying how the body uses food, we can choose foods that lead to wellness.

Have You Ever Wondered ?

▼ Spaghetti can give your body energy. Why?
▼ Food labels can help you make wise decisions. How?
▼ If you must lose weight, you should try to lose weight slowly. Why?

As you read this unit, think about your own eating habits. Think about making decisions for choosing healthy foods for good health.

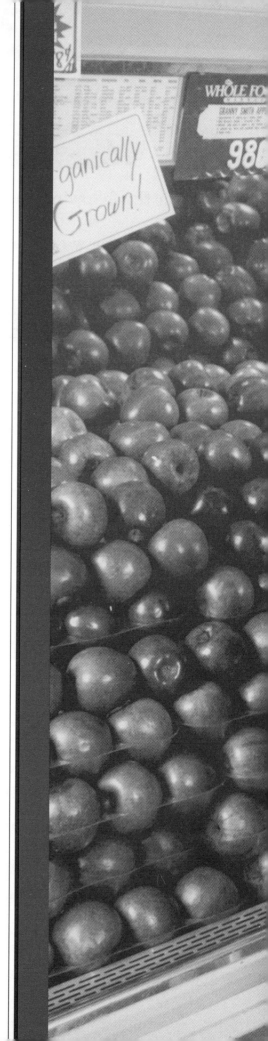

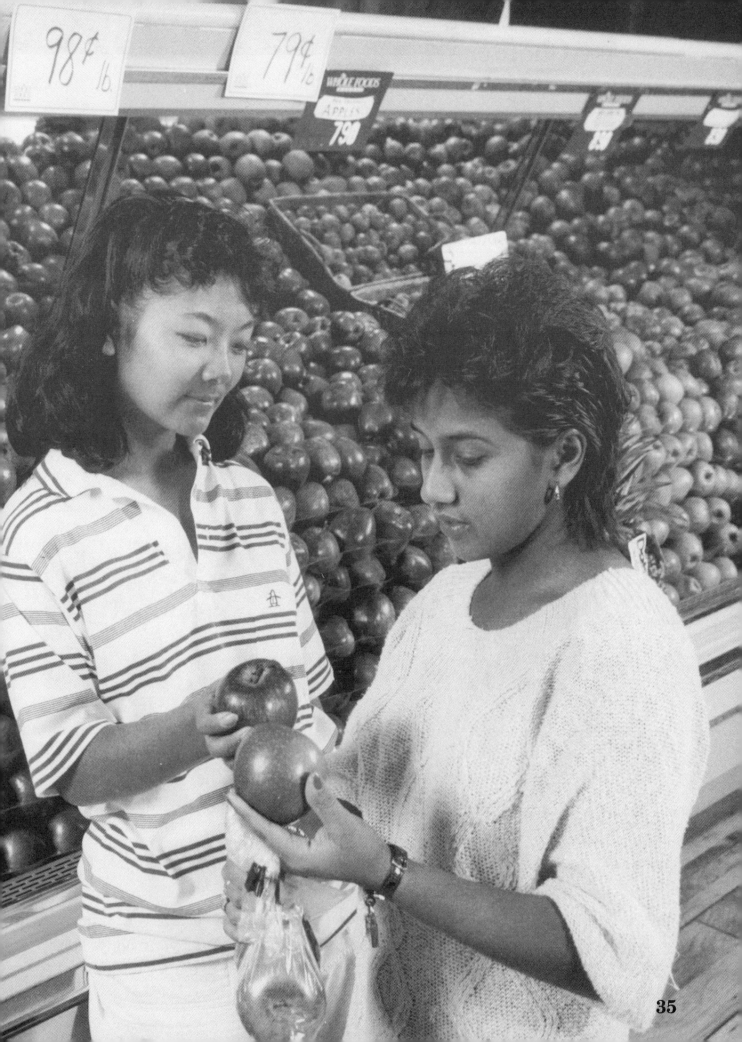

98¢ lb.   79¢ lb.

APPLES 79¢

35

Chapter 5

Choosing Healthy Foods

Think About as You Read

- **Why do you need food?**
- **Why do you need calories?**
- **How do nutrients help your body?**

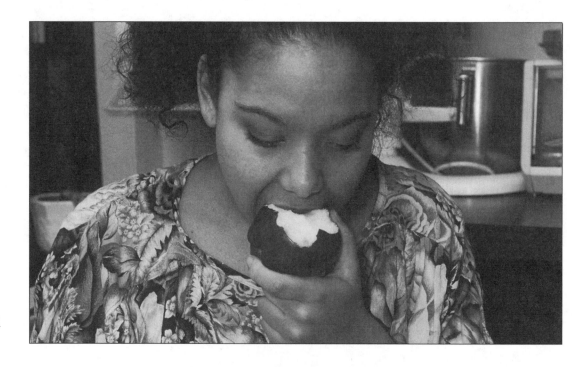

Choosing healthy foods to eat leads to good health and wellness.

Do you like to eat a snack when you come home from school? Most students do. Think about your snacks. Are they fruits or vegetables? Are they chips or candy? Some foods are healthier than others. By studying **nutrition** you can learn to make healthy food choices. Choosing healthy foods leads to good health and wellness.

Nutrition is the food needed by the body for life and growth.

Calories and Food

The food you eat provides energy for your body. Your body uses energy all the time. You use a lot of energy when you run or swim. You need less energy for sleeping and talking.

The energy in food is measured in **calories**. Different foods contain different amounts of calories. An apple has about 80 calories. A cup of ice cream has about 300 calories.

Different people need different amounts of calories. A person who plays sports needs more calories than a person who never exercises. You need more calories when you are sick than when you are not sick. During the teen years, bodies need energy to grow and change. So teen-agers may need more calories than most adults. People gain weight when they eat more calories than their bodies use for energy.

Why Do You Need Nutrients?

The food you eat also provides **nutrients** for your body. You need six kinds of nutrients for good health.

Three kinds of nutrients provide the body with calories. **Carbohydrates**, **proteins**, and fats are nutrients that provide calories. **Vitamins**, **minerals**, and water are three nutrients that do not provide calories.

Nutrients are substances in food that the body needs for health and life.

Carbohydrates are nutrients that give the body energy.

Proteins are nutrients that the body uses for growth and repair.

Vitamins are a group of nutrients that the body must have in small amounts in order to work and grow as it should.

Minerals are nutrients that are needed by the body to provide healthy teeth, muscles, bones, and blood cells.

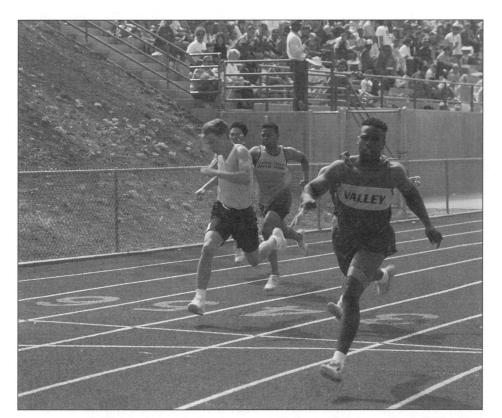

You need many calories when you play sports because you use a lot of energy.

How Do Nutrients Help Your Body?

Each of the six kinds of nutrients helps the body in a different way. The chart on page 39 has information about each nutrient. Let's find out why each kind is important.

1. <u>Carbohydrates</u> are our most important source of energy. There are three types of carbohydrates. Sugar provides quick energy. **Starch** provides longer-lasting energy. Bread, rice, and cereals are three starches. Most of your calories should come from starches. **Fiber** helps you get rid of body wastes. Fruits, vegetables, and whole grains have fiber.

2. <u>Proteins</u> contain **amino acids**. Amino acids help the body grow. They also help the body repair itself. Foods like meat, fish, and milk are complete proteins. Each of these foods contains all the amino acids that the body needs. Other foods contain only some of the amino acids. But you can get all the proteins you need by eating a few foods with different amino acids. By eating beans and rice or macaroni and cheese, you will get all the amino acids you need.

3. <u>Fats</u> are another source of energy. They contain many more calories than carbohydrates or proteins. You need only very small amounts of fat from the food you eat.

Fiber is a carbohydrate from plants that helps the body remove wastes but does not become part of the body cells. The fiber in a food has no calories.

Amino acids are substances that make up proteins.

Most of your calories should come from carbohydrates such as fruits and vegetables.

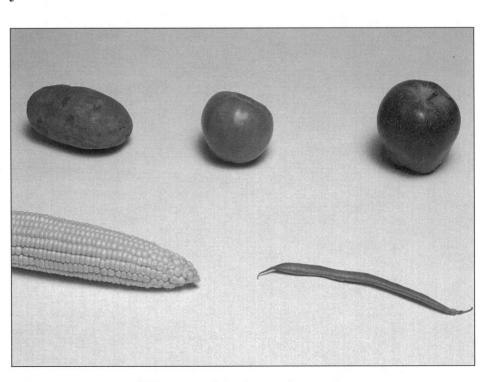

38

THE SIX KINDS OF NUTRIENTS YOUR BODY NEEDS

Nutrient	How does the nutrient help your body?	What foods have this nutrient?
1 Carbohydrates		
Sugar	gives the body quick energy	white sugar, brown sugar, honey, syrup, candy, fruit
Starch	gives the body longer-lasting energy	potatoes, rice, cereals, corn, noodles, bread, sweet potatoes, barley, pasta
Fiber	helps the body remove wastes	fruits and vegetables with skins, whole grains (brown rice, oatmeal, whole wheat bread), plain popcorn
2 Proteins	help build muscles, bones, and teeth help the body make new cells	meat, fish, chicken, eggs, turkey, milk, cheese, peanut butter, beans
3 Fats	give the body energy keep the body warm	butter, margarine, mayonnaise, peanut butter, oils, fatty meat, whole milk, cheese
4 Minerals		
Iron	helps red blood cells carry oxygen	red meat, beans, dark green vegetables, whole grains
Calcium	helps build strong bones and teeth	milk, cheese, peas, beans, broccoli, spinach, green vegetables, salmon, sardines
5 Vitamins		
Vitamin A	helps you see in the dark helps build healthy skin and teeth	carrots, green vegetables, fruits, butter, cream, whole milk, cheese
Vitamin B_1	helps keep the brain and nerve cells healthy	brown rice, whole grains, cereals, milk, meat, fish, eggs, potatoes
Vitamin B_2	helps keep the skin healthy	milk, cereal, whole grains, cheese, meat, eggs, fish, chicken
Vitamin C	helps keep skin, gums, and bones healthy	tomatoes, oranges, lemons, grapefruits, melons, potatoes, green vegetables
Vitamin D	helps build strong bones and teeth	eggs, milk, butter, fish, oils
6 Water	helps the body digest food and get rid of wastes	water, milk, juice

Eating foods that have too much fat causes you to gain weight. People who eat many foods that provide fats often have too much **cholesterol** in their blood. Too much cholesterol in the blood can cause heart disease. Fatty meats, butter, whole milk, hard cheese, and egg yolks are high in cholesterol. You should eat only small amounts of these foods. Instead eat foods like fish, skinless chicken, egg whites, and skim milk.

4. Minerals help the body grow and work well. You need only very small amounts of different minerals from the food you eat each day. The chart on page 39 tells you about two important minerals.

5. Vitamins help the body stay healthy. There are 13 different kinds of vitamins. You should get all of your vitamins from food. People who have a healthy **diet** do not need vitamin pills. The chart on page 39 tells you about five important vitamins.

6. Water helps your body in many ways. It helps keep your body at the right temperature. It helps remove wastes from your body. The water in your blood carries nutrients to every part of your body. You should drink six to eight glasses of water each day.

To look and feel your best, eat foods that provide enough nutrients and calories for your body. In the next chapter, you will learn how to plan a healthy diet.

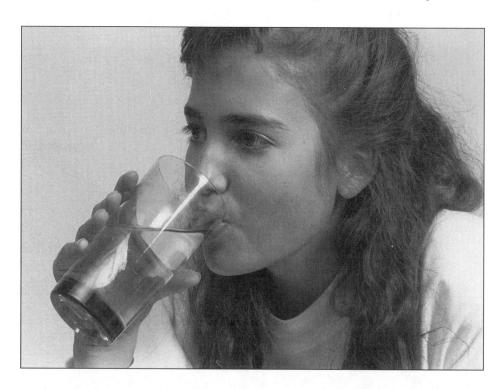

You should drink six to eight glasses of water a day.

Using What You Learned

Vocabulary—Matching

Match each vocabulary word in **Group B** with a sentence from **Group A** that tells about the word. Write the letter of the correct answer on your paper.

Group A

1. The energy in food is measured in these.

2. This carbohydrate helps you get rid of body wastes.

3. Too much of this in your blood can cause heart disease.

4. You study this so you can make healthy food choices.

5. Your body needs six kinds of these from the foods you eat.

6. This carbohydrate gives your body longer-lasting energy than sugar.

7. These nutrients contain amino acids.

Group B

a. cholesterol

b. nutrients

c. starch

d. fiber

e. calories

f. proteins

g. nutrition

Comprehension—True or False

Write **True** on your paper for each sentence that is true. Write **False** on your paper for each sentence that is false. There are four false sentences. Rewrite the false sentences on your paper to make them true.

1. Your body does not use energy when you sleep.

2. Fats are the most important source of energy.

3. Each person's body needs a different number of calories.

4. Most of your calories should come from water.

5. You do not need vitamin pills if you make healthy food choices.

6. Choosing healthy foods helps you to reach your goal of wellness.

7. The nutrients in honey and syrup give you quick energy.

8. Calcium is a mineral that helps red blood cells carry oxygen.

9. Fats are found in fatty meats, butter, whole milk, cheese, and peanut butter.

10. Water helps keep your body at the right temperature.

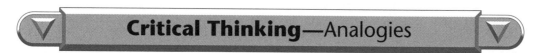

Critical Thinking—Analogies

An **analogy** compares two pairs of words. The words in the first pair are alike in the same way as the words in the second pair. For example, **fruit** is to **fiber** as **candy** is to **sugar.** Number your paper from 1 to 6. Use a word or words in the box to finish each sentence. Write the correct answers on your paper.

cholesterol	sugar	nutrients
calories	amino acids	calcium

1. Pounds are to weight as _____ are to energy.

2. Food is to energy as _____ are to good health.

3. Fats are to weight as _____ is to heart disease.

4. Proteins are to body growth as _____ is to quick energy.

5. Nutrients are to food as _____ are to proteins.

6. Vitamin C is to oranges as _____ is to milk.

Decision Making for Nutrition

Think About as You Read

- Why do we need to eat from the food groups?
- What should you eat in restaurants?
- What can you learn by reading food labels?

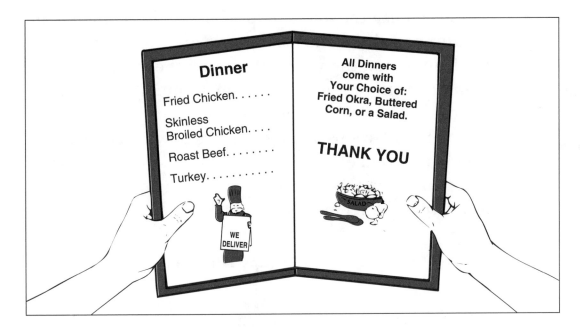

Choose healthy foods when you eat in restaurants. The foods you choose should be low in fat and salt.

José ate dinner in a restaurant. He decided to order skinless, **broiled** chicken and salad. José chose foods that have protein, carbohydrates, and vitamins. His food choices are low in fat, cholesterol, salt, and calories. José had made a decision for wellness.

Food that is **broiled** is cooked over an open flame or under the flame in the broiler of an oven.

Seven Rules for a Healthy Diet

The American **Cancer** Society believes that seven diet rules can help protect you from cancer and heart disease.

1. Eat different kinds of food. Include foods that have carbohydrates with starch and fiber.

Cancer is a disease in which unhealthy cells multiply too rapidly and destroy healthy body parts.

Blood pressure is the pressure of the blood as it moves against the walls of the body's blood vessels.

Smoked foods are prepared for future use by using smoke. Bacon is a food that is sometimes smoked.

Nitrites are chemicals that are added to certain fish and meats, such as hot dogs and sliced sandwich meats. Nitrites may be harmful to health.

A **balanced diet** means eating enough servings from each of the food groups. A balanced diet provides the right amount of calories and nutrients.

2. Eat the right amount of calories to keep your body at a healthy weight.
3. Eat lots of fiber.
4. Eat much less fat.
5. Eat less sugar and salt. People gain weight from sugar because it is high in calories. Too much salt causes high **blood pressure** in many people. This can lead to heart disease.
6. Avoid **smoked** foods and foods with **nitrites**.
7. Don't drink alcohol. Alcohol damages the body. It has no nutrients, and it has many calories.

Plan Your Diet Around the Food Groups

You can use the food groups chart on page 45 to plan a **balanced diet**. The food groups are the grain group; the fruit group; the vegetable group; the milk group; and the meat, egg, nut, and bean group. The chart lists the healthiest foods in each group.

The Food Groups Triangle shows how much food you should eat from each food group. Eat more foods from the groups near the bottom of the triangle. Eat less foods from the groups at the top.

Use the Food Groups Triangle to plan a balanced diet.

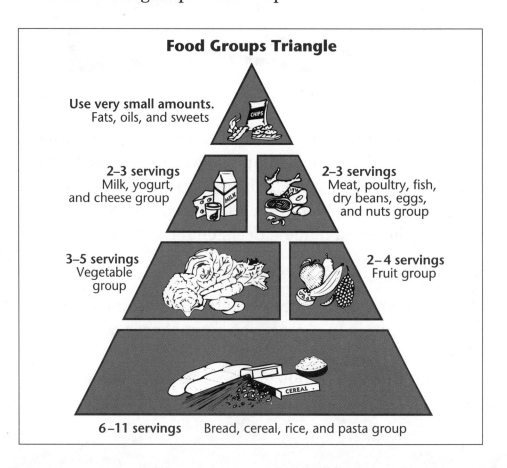

Food Groups Triangle

Use very small amounts.
Fats, oils, and sweets

2–3 servings
Milk, yogurt, and cheese group

2–3 servings
Meat, poultry, fish, dry beans, eggs, and nuts group

3–5 servings
Vegetable group

2–4 servings
Fruit group

6–11 servings   Bread, cereal, rice, and pasta group

44

Food Groups

Group	Foods in This Group	Foods to Avoid	Healthy Choices
1. Grain Group Eat 6 to 11 servings each day.	bread, cereal, pasta, rice, barley	sweet cereals, pasta in oily sauce, cakes, cookies	whole wheat bread, whole grain cereal, brown rice, bagels
2. Fruit Group Eat 2 to 4 servings each day.	all fruits, fruit juice	canned fruit in heavy syrup	different kinds of fresh fruits
3. Vegetable Group Eat 3 to 5 servings each day.	all vegetables	fried vegetables	fresh salads; different kinds of fresh, frozen, or canned vegetables
4. Meat-Nut-Eggs-Bean Group Eat 2 to 3 servings each day.	chicken, turkey, meat, fish, eggs, dried beans, peanut butter	smoked meats and fish, lunch meats with nitrites, bacon, fatty meats, hot dogs, egg yolks, chicken skin, canned tuna in oil	skinless chicken, turkey, egg whites, lean meat, small portions of fish, canned tuna in water
5. Milk Group Teen-agers need 3 servings each day.	milk, cheese, ice cream, yogurt	cream, butter, hard cheese, whole milk, ice cream	skim milk, 1% low-fat milk, low-fat cheese, corn oil margarine, low-fat frozen ice cream and yogurt
6. High-Calorie Snack Group Avoid these snack foods.	chips, candy, cookies, salted peanuts, pies	sweet and fatty snacks	fruit, raw vegetables, unbuttered popcorn, unsalted pretzels, rice cakes

Try to eat the correct number of servings from each of the five food groups every day. You must also drink six to eight glasses of water each day.

There is a sixth food group on the chart. It is the high-calorie snack group. The foods in this group are often high in fat, sugar, or salt. They have few nutrients. Try not to eat these snacks often.

Healthy Meals in Restaurants

Many foods in fast-food restaurants are salty and fried. The food is often high in calories.

How can you eat healthy foods in restaurants? Choose lean meats or chicken. Always remove the skin from your chicken. Choose foods that are baked or broiled. Avoid fried foods. Choose low-fat frozen **yogurt** instead of milk shakes. Choose corn on the cob instead of French fries. Order a fresh salad but use only a small amount of salad dressing. Many salad dressings are high in fat, salt, and cholesterol.

Yogurt is a thick, soft food made from milk.

Food Labels

Most foods that are packed in cans, boxes, and bags

This food label tells you that Cereal Flakes has no fat, many vitamins, and too much sugar.

Cereal Flakes

Nutrition Facts

Serving Size 3/4 Cup (30g)
Servings per Container 14

Amount Per Serving	Cereal	Cereal with 1/2 Cup Skim Milk
Calories	120	160
Calories from Fat	0	0
	% Daily Value**	
Total Fat 0g*	**0%**	**0%**
Saturated Fat 0g	**0%**	**0%**
Cholesterol 0mg	**0%**	**0%**
Sodium 200mg	**8%**	**11%**
Potassium 20mg	**1%**	**6%**
Total Carbohydrate 28g	**9%**	**11%**
Dietary Fiber 0g	**0%**	**0%**
Sugars 13g		
Other Carbohydrate 15g		
Protein 1g		
Vitamin A	15%	20%
Vitamin C	25%	25%
Calcium	0%	15%
Iron	25%	25%
Vitamin D	10%	25%

		% Daily Value**
Thiamin	25%	30%
Riboflavin	25%	35%
Niacin	25%	25%
Vitamin B6	25%	25%
Folate	25%	25%

* Amount in cereal. One serving of cereal with one half cup of skim milk provides 265mg sodium, 34g total carbohydrate (19g sugars), and 5g protein.

** Percent Daily Values are based on a 2,000 calorie diet. Your daily values may be higher or lower depending on your calorie needs:

	Calories	2,000	2,500
Total Fat	Less than	65g	80g
Sat. Fat	Less than	20g	25g
Cholesterol	Less than	300mg	300mg
Sodium	Less than	2,400mg	2,400mg
Potassium		3,500mg	3,500mg
Total Carbohydrate		300g	375g
Dietary Fiber		25g	30g

Ingredients: Corn, sugar, salt, malt flavoring, corn syrup

Vitamins and Iron: Ascorbic acid (vitamin C), niacinamide, iron, pyridoxine hydrochloride (vitamin B6), riboflavin (vitamin B2), vitamin A palmitate (protected with BHT), thiamin hydrochloride (vitamin B1), folic acid, and vitamin D

Cold Oat Cereal

Nutrition Facts

Serving Size   1 cup (30g)
Servings Per Container   14

Amount Per Serving	Cereal	Cereal with 1/2 Cup Skim Milk
Calories	110	150
Calories from Fat	15	20
	% Daily Value**	
Total Fat 2g*	3%	3%
Saturated Fat 0g	0%	2%
Cholesterol 0mg	0%	1%
Sodium 280mg	12%	14%
Potassium 90mg	3%	8%
Total Carbohydrate 23g	8%	10%
Dietary Fiber 3g	11%	11%
Sugars 1g		
Other Carbohydrate 19g		
Protein 3g		
Vitamin A	25%	30%
Vitamin C	25%	25%
Calcium	4%	20%
Iron	45%	45%
Vitamin D	10%	25%
Thiamin	25%	30%
Riboflavin	25%	35%
Niacin	25%	25%

	% Daily Value**	
Vitamin B6	25%	25%
Folic Acid	25%	25%
Phosphorus	10%	25%
Magnesium	8%	10%
Zinc	25%	30%
Copper	4%	4%

* Amount in cereal. One serving of cereal with one half cup of skim milk provides 2g fat (0.5g saturated fat), less than 5mg cholesterol, 350mg sodium, 29g total carbohydrate (7g sugars) and 7g protein.

** Percent Daily Values are based on a 2,000 calorie diet. Your daily values may be higher or lower depending on your calorie needs:

	Calories:	2,000	2,500
Total Fat	Less than	65g	80g
Sat. Fat	Less than	20g	25g
Cholesterol	Less than	300mg	300mg
Sodium	Less than	2,400mg	2,400mg
Potassium		3,500mg	3,500mg
Total Carbohydrate		300g	375g
Dietary Fiber		25g	30g

Ingredients: Whole oat flour (includes the oat bran), modified food starch, wheat starch, sugar, salt, oat fiber, trisodium phosphate, calcium carbonate, vitamin E (mixed tocopherols) added to preserve freshness

Vitamins and Minerals: Vitamin C (sodium ascorbate), iron and zinc (mineral nutrients), A B vitamin (niacin), vitamin B6 (pyridoxine hydrochloride), vitamin A (palmitate), vitamin B2 (riboflavin), vitamin B1 (thiamin mono-nitrate), A B vitamin (folic acid), vitamin D

This food label tells you that Cold Oat Cereal has a lot of fiber and iron. It has very little sugar.

have food labels. Labels tell about the food's nutrients and calories. They list the **ingredients** in a food.

Ingredients are listed in order of weight from most to least. The label for Cereal Flakes on page 46 shows that the first ingredient is corn. This cereal has more corn than any other ingredient.

A food label lists the serving size. The label also tells you how many calories and nutrients are in a serving. The Cold Oat Cereal label says that one cup of cereal provides 110 calories. So if you eat two cups of cereal, you will be eating 220 calories.

Food labels can help you choose healthy foods. Read the cereal label on this page. Cold Oat Cereal has a lot of healthy fiber and iron. It only has one **gram** of sugar, while Cereal Flakes has 13 grams of sugar. From these labels we can decide that Cold Oat Cereal is the healthier choice.

Use what you have learned about nutrition to plan your diet. A balanced diet will help you have wellness.

Ingredients are the parts of a food that are mixed with others when cooking, baking, or packaging.

Grams are measures of weight.

Using What You Learned

Vocabulary—Find the Meaning

Write on your paper the word or words that best complete each sentence.

1. Eating too much salt can cause high _____ .

   wellness   **blood pressure**   **fiber**

2. It is best to avoid foods with chemicals called _____ .

   yogurt   **starches**   **nitrites**

3. Eating the right number of servings from each of the food groups gives you a _____ .

   food label   **balanced diet**   **heart disease**

4. Labels tell a food's nutrients, calories, and _____ .

   ingredients   **restaurant**   **quality**

5. A healthy diet can help protect you from heart disease and _____ .

   cancer   **alcohol**   **food groups**

6. You should avoid foods that are _____ if you want to protect yourself from cancer.

   vegetables   **canned in water**   **smoked**

Comprehension—Write the Answer

Write a sentence on your paper to answer each question.

1. Why should you eat less sugar?

2. What can cause high blood pressure?

3. Where should you look to find out about a food's ingredients?

4. How can you be sure to have a balanced diet?

5. How many glasses of water should you drink each day?

6. Why should you avoid foods in the high-calorie snack group?

7. From which food group should you eat the most servings each day?

Critical Thinking—Cause and Effect

Write sentences on your paper by matching each cause on the left with an effect on the right.

Cause

1. You always read the labels on packaged foods, so _____

2. You believe you can help protect yourself from cancer and heart disease, so _____

3. You eat too much salt, so _____

4. You eat the right number of calories, so _____

5. You plan a balanced diet, so _____

6. Many salad dressings are high in fat, salt, and cholesterol, so _____

7. You want to eat a healthy dessert, so _____

Effect

a. you eat the correct number of servings from each food group.

b. your body stays at a healthy weight.

c. you order a salad without salad dressing.

d. you know what ingredients the foods contain.

e. you follow the American Cancer Society's seven diet rules.

f. you choose low-fat frozen yogurt.

g. your blood pressure may go up.

Chapter 7

Controlling Your Weight

Think About as You Read

- Why should growing teen-agers gain weight?
- How can people lose or gain weight safely?
- Why are eating disorders dangerous?

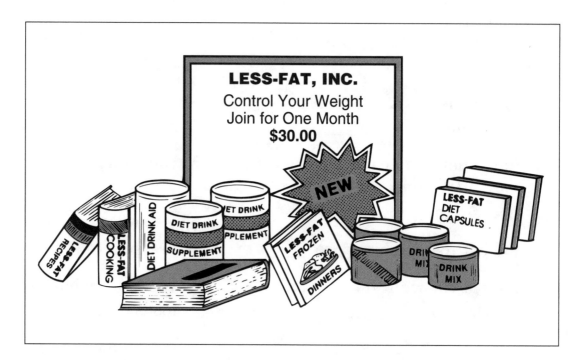

LESS-FAT, INC.
Control Your Weight
Join for One Month
$30.00

NEW

LESS-FAT RECIPES

LESS-FAT COOKING

DIET DRINK AID

DIET DRINK SUPPLEMENT

DIET DRINK SUPPLEMENT

LESS-FAT FROZEN DINNERS

DRINK MIX

DRINK MIX

LESS-FAT DIET CAPSULES

People try many different diet foods and diets in order to lose weight.

Every year millions of Americans go on diets to lose weight. Some diets are very low in calories. Other diets are very expensive because people must join a special diet group. Sometimes they must buy special diet foods. Some of these diets are dangerous. They do not provide all the nutrients people need.

Diets and Weight Control

Most people go on a diet because they are overweight. They want to lose weight. Underweight people go on diets to gain weight.

50

Each person has an **ideal weight**. A tall person with large bones should weigh more than a short person with small bones. During the teen years, the body is growing and changing. It is healthy for teen-agers to gain weight while their bodies are growing. Your doctor or school nurse can tell you what weight is right for you.

Two people who are the same height can have different ideal weights. Carlos and Tom are the same height. Carlos has larger bones and muscles than Tom. So Carlos weighs more than Tom. But both boys have the right weight for their height.

To reach the goal of wellness, work at keeping your ideal weight. Being overweight can cause heart disease and other diseases. So controlling your weight helps your physical health. It also helps your emotional health. People feel good about their appearance when they control their weight. This helps their self-esteem. It helps them feel accepted by others.

People who are underweight can work at gaining weight. To gain weight, eat more calories than your body needs for energy. If you want to gain weight, try to eat 500 extra calories each day. Get more sleep. You use fewer calories when you sleep. Do more exercise. Exercise makes your muscles larger. You weigh more when you have larger muscles.

Your **ideal weight** is the weight that is right for someone of your age, height, and bone size.

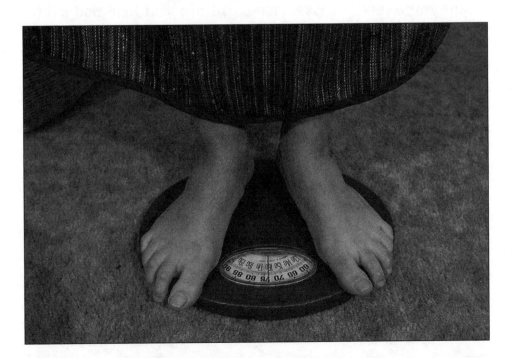

Controlling your weight helps your physical health. It also helps your self-esteem.

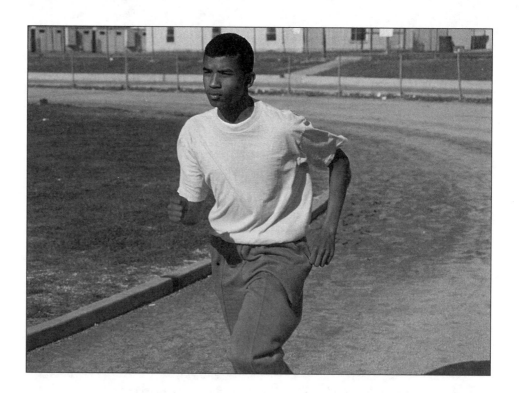

Your body uses more calories when you exercise. Exercising helps you lose weight.

To lose weight, eat fewer calories than your body needs for energy. Since you will not get enough energy from food, your body must use its own fat for energy. Then you will lose weight by losing body fat.

What else can people do to lose body fat safely? Eat less food. Eat low-fat, balanced meals. Drink six to eight glasses of water each day. Always eat breakfast, lunch, and dinner. People get very hungry when they miss meals. Then they eat more calories than they need. Exercise more. Your body uses more calories when you exercise. Exercise can help you lose body fat. Before starting your diet, discuss it with your doctor or school nurse. They can help you plan a safe diet.

It is best to lose weight slowly. You should not lose more than two pounds in one week. People must learn new, healthy eating habits to lose weight and not gain it back. These healthy habits will help them control their weight throughout life.

Eating Disorders

People with **eating disorders** are afraid of gaining weight. Eating disorders cause very unhealthy eating habits that harm the body.

Some people have a terrible fear of becoming overweight. This fear can cause **eating disorders**. Eating disorders sometimes lead to death.

Anorexia nervosa and **bulimia** are two eating disorders. Boys can have these disorders. But most people with these disorders are teen-age girls.

People with anorexia nervosa have a great fear of being overweight. So they starve themselves. They eat only very small amounts of food. They often **vomit** after eating in order to get food out of their bodies. These people try to be thinner and thinner. They don't get enough calories and nutrients. Sometimes they starve to death.

People with bulimia do **binge** eating. They eat huge amounts of food at one time. Then they vomit to get rid of the food. Sometimes they starve themselves after a binge. Bulimia harms the body. **Acids** in vomit damage the teeth and throat. People with bulimia do not get enough nutrients.

People with eating disorders have poor emotional health. They have low self-esteem. They do not accept themselves. They need help to solve their problems. People with eating disorders should ask for help from their school nurse or doctor.

Controlling your weight helps you reach the goal of wellness. Healthy, low-fat meals and exercise can help you control your weight. Controlling your weight helps your physical and emotional health.

To **vomit** is to throw up food from the stomach.

An **acid** is a chemical with a sour taste.

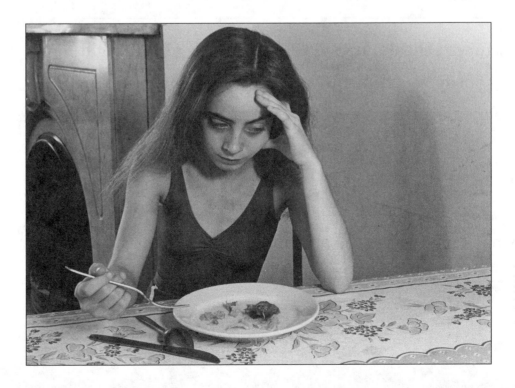

People with anorexia nervosa think they are too heavy. These people are afraid to eat.

53

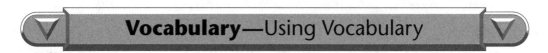

Vocabulary—Using Vocabulary

Use the word or words to write a complete sentence on your paper about weight control.

1. binge
2. ideal weight
3. anorexia nervosa
4. bulimia
5. calories
6. exercise

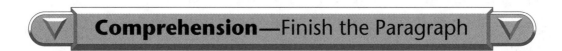

Comprehension—Finish the Paragraph

Number your paper from 1 to 10. Use a word from the box to finish each sentence. Write the correct answers on your paper.

exercises	calories	ideal	control	energy
overweight	meals	more	nutrients	weight

Check with your doctor or school nurse to find out what __(1)__ is right for you. Keeping your __(2)__ body weight helps you reach your goal of wellness.

You might need to plan a diet to __(3)__ your weight. Your doctor or school nurse can help you plan a safe diet. The diet you choose must have all the __(4)__ your body needs.

If you are underweight, you can gain weight by eating more __(5)__ than your body needs. You may need to increase the amount of sleep you get in order to gain weight. Doing __(6)__ to build larger muscles can help you gain weight, too.

You may need to lose weight if you are __(7)__ . You can do this by eating fewer calories than your body needs for __(8)__ . Plan low-fat, balanced __(9)__ . Exercise can also help you lose body fat because your body uses __(10)__ calories.

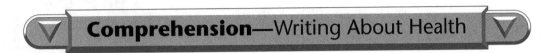

Comprehension—Writing About Health

Answer the following question in complete sentences on your paper.

How can keeping your ideal weight help your physical and emotional health?

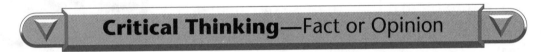

Critical Thinking—Fact or Opinion

Write **Fact** on your paper for each fact below. Write **Opinion** for each opinion. You should find four sentences that are opinions.

1. Some diets do not have all the nutrients your body needs.

2. Your ideal weight might be different than your friend's, even if you are both the same height.

3. People always need to lose weight.

4. Teen-agers never need to gain weight.

5. Heart disease and other diseases can be caused by being overweight.

6. Eating more calories than your body needs can help you gain weight.

7. Teen-agers can eat as many calories as they want and never gain weight.

8. Skipping meals is the best way to lose body fat safely.

9. Increasing your exercise can help you lose weight.

10. Healthy eating habits can help you control your weight throughout your life.

UNIT 4

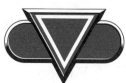

Personal Health

Imagine you are going to a special party. You want to look your best. So you spend extra time getting ready. You look in the mirror a few times to be sure you look just right.

To look our best on special days, we must take care of ourselves every day. To look and feel our best we need good personal health habits. We must learn how to keep our bodies strong and fit. We must care for our skin, hair, and teeth. Our eyes and ears need good care, too.

Have You Ever Wondered ?

▼ Your body needs exercise at least three times a week. What kind of exercise?
▼ The sun can damage your skin. How?
▼ Healthy teeth can help you have good health. How?
▼ Soft music is better for your ears than loud music. Why?

As you read this unit, you will learn how to care for your personal health. You will learn how good personal health habits can help you reach the goal of wellness.

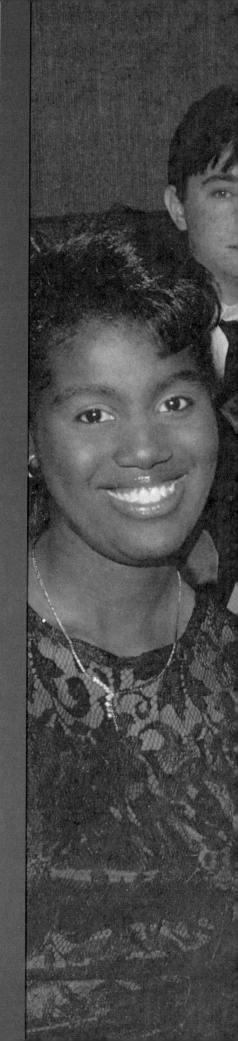

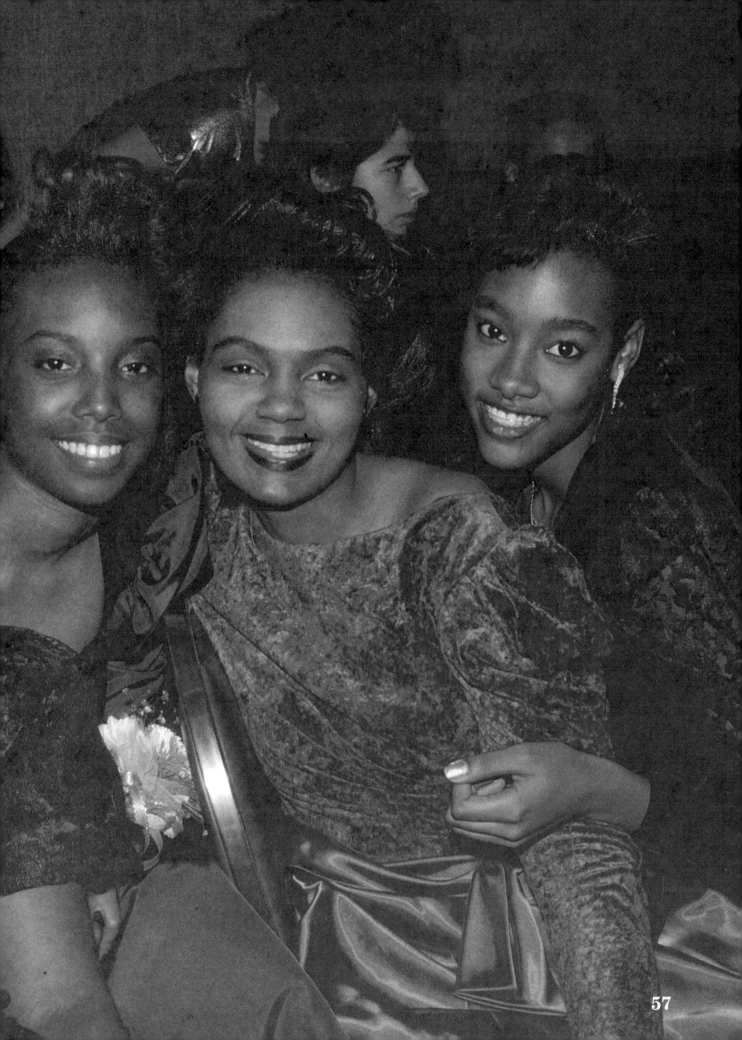

Chapter 8

Physical Fitness

Think About as You Read

- How does exercise help your physical, emotional, and social health?
- What three fitness areas should your exercise program try to improve?
- What kinds of exercise do you need in a fitness program?

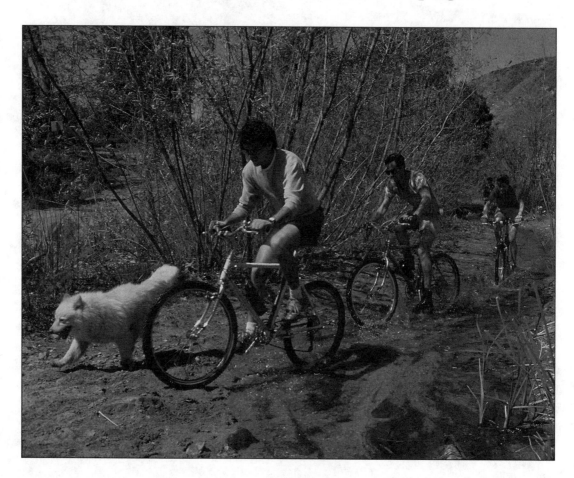

Physical fitness through exercise helps you reach the goal of wellness.

You have good **physical fitness** when you can use your body to work, exercise, and play without getting tired quickly.

Matthew is always busy. He plays on the school football team. He has homework every day. He works at a part-time job once a week. But Matthew takes time for **physical fitness**. He exercises three times a week. He knows that physical fitness is important.

58

Physical Fitness and Wellness

Physical fitness through exercise helps your physical health in many ways. It helps your **cardiovascular system**. It does this by making your heart stronger. Exercise also keeps the blood vessels called **arteries** healthy. Exercise helps lower the amount of cholesterol in the blood. It also helps people control their weight. People who are physically fit often have lower blood pressure than people who are not fit. People who are physically fit usually have less chance of getting heart disease.

Exercise helps your physical health in three other ways. It helps you build strong muscles. It helps you have better **posture** and strong bones. Building strong bones helps protect you from **osteoporosis**. Eating foods with calcium also builds strong bones.

Exercise helps your emotional health. Exercising helps you feel less stress. It also helps you control your weight. It helps you have good posture. This helps you look your best. Feeling good about the way you look raises your self-esteem.

Exercise helps your social health, too. Bike riding and swimming are fun sports. Your friends or family can join you in these sports. Team sports, like baseball, help you learn to get along with a group.

Your **cardiovascular system** includes your heart, blood vessels, and blood. This system brings oxygen and nutrients to all parts of your body.

Your **arteries** are tubes that carry blood from your heart to different body parts.

Your **posture** is the way you carry your body when sitting and standing.

Osteoporosis is a problem in which the bones lose calcium. As a result the bones become weaker and break easily.

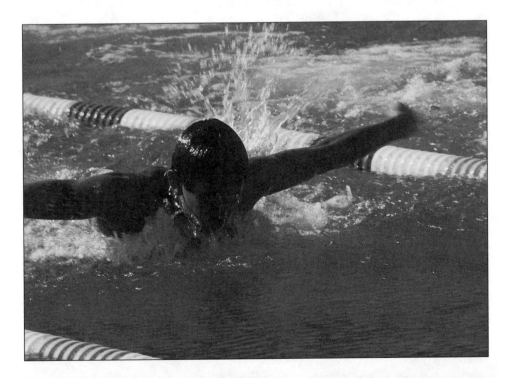

Exercises like swimming help your heart and your posture. They are also fun.

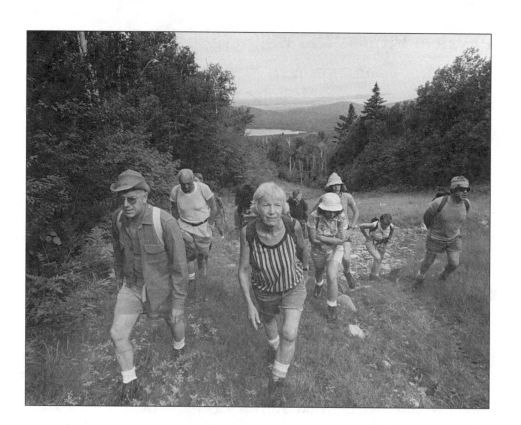

People of all age groups can enjoy sports like walking, swimming, skating, and tennis.

Planning a Personal Exercise Program

Plan your own physical fitness program with exercises that you enjoy. If you enjoy your activities, you will do them more often. Choose exercises that you can enjoy all your life. Walking, skating, swimming, and tennis are some of the sports that are enjoyed by all age groups.

Allow time for physical fitness. Exercise at least three times each week. Exercise for at least 30 minutes each time.

Your exercises should build three physical fitness areas. These areas are **endurance**, strength, and **flexibility**.

You have **endurance** when you can do activities, like running, for a long period of time.

An **aerobic** exercise helps the heart become stronger.

Endurance helps you build a strong cardiovascular system. **Aerobic** exercises like running and jumping rope build endurance.

You must build muscles to have physical strength. Pushups and pull-ups build strong muscles. Lifting weights also builds strength.

Flexibility helps you to stretch your body in many directions. Stretching exercises build flexibility.

60

Planning a Home Exercise Program

An exercise program should have three parts.

1. The warm-up. Do exercises that stretch your muscles for five to ten minutes. The warm-up prepares your heart and other muscles for more exercise.

2. The **workout**. Do at least 15 minutes of aerobic exercise. Running, aerobic dancing, and jumping rope are aerobic exercises. Also try to use small arm and leg weights. They will help you build muscle strength.

3. The cool-down. Repeat the warm-up exercises. Do them for five to ten minutes. This helps your heart slow down. Then your body can relax.

Build your physical fitness slowly. For example, the first week Linda did only 10 sit-ups each time she exercised. After a week she did 15. After two weeks she did 20.

Make physical fitness part of your life. It will help improve your physical, emotional, and social health. This will help you reach your goal of wellness.

A **workout** is a group of exercises that helps make the heart and other muscles stronger.

Your Three-Part Exercise Program

The Warm-up	The Workout	The Cool-down
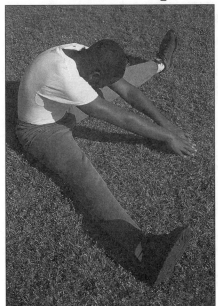	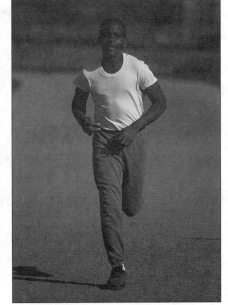	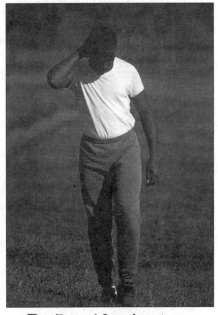
Do 5 to 10 minutes of stretching.	Do one or more aerobic exercises for at least 15 minutes.	Do 5 to 10 minutes of stretching.

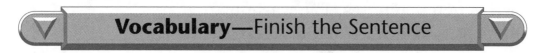
Vocabulary—Finish the Sentence

Choose a word from the box to complete each sentence. Write the correct answers on your paper.

osteoporosis	aerobic	cardiovascular
flexibility	posture	workout

1. Exercise helps your _____ system.

2. The second part of an exercise program is the _____ .

3. The way you carry your body is your _____ .

4. Swimming is an _____ exercise.

5. Building strong bones through exercise helps protect you from _____ .

6. Good _____ helps you to stretch your body in many directions.

Comprehension—True or False

Write **True** on your paper for each sentence that is true. Write **False** on your paper for each sentence that is false. There are four false sentences. Rewrite the false sentences on your paper to make them true.

1. Exercise helps your social health.

2. An exercise program should only develop endurance.

3. People who are physically fit have a greater chance of having high blood pressure.

4. It is important to build physical fitness slowly.

5. Exercise helps you build strong muscles.

6. Having good posture helps you look your best.

7. Joining team sports can help you learn to get along with a group.

8. You should plan a physical fitness program with exercises you find difficult to do.

9. You can build physical strength by lifting weights.

10. Stretching exercises limit your flexibility.

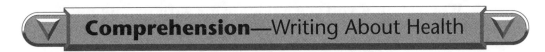

Comprehension—Writing About Health

Answer the following question in complete sentences on your paper.

How does exercise help your emotional health?

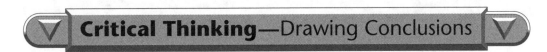

Critical Thinking—Drawing Conclusions

Read the paragraph. Then use the six steps below to decide what to do about improving physical fitness. Write complete sentences on your paper to answer each question.

Imagine that you want to lose weight. You decide to improve your physical fitness to reach this goal. You are developing a home exercise program for yourself. You do not enjoy exercising by yourself, but no one wants to exercise with you.

Step 1. What is the problem?

Step 2. What are two ways to solve the problem?

Step 3. What is one consequence for each choice listed in Step 2?

Step 4. Which choice do you think is best?

Step 5. What can you do to put your decision into action?

Step 6. Think about your decision. Why was this the best choice for you?

The Care of Skin, Hair, and Nails

Think About as You Read

- How can you take care of acne?
- How do you protect your skin from the sun?
- When should you see a doctor for skin problems?

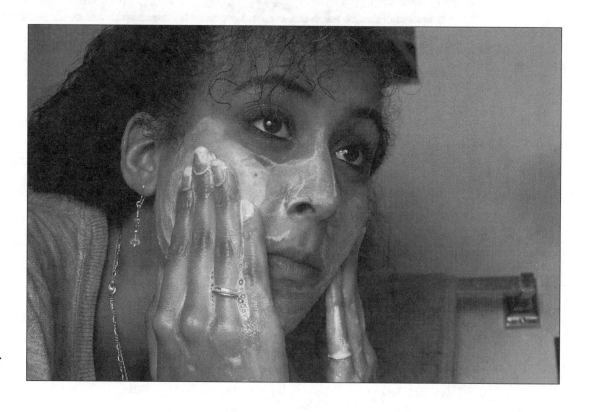

To care for your skin, wash your face twice a day. Use warm water and soap.

Lisa is unhappy. Her hair and skin have changed during the past few years. Her hair is oily. She has pimples on her face. How should Lisa care for her hair and skin?

Acne and Other Skin Problems

Bacteria are very tiny living things that can sometimes cause you to become sick.

The skin covering your body protects you. It keeps **bacteria** out of your body. Your skin keeps your body temperature from becoming too hot or too cold.

Your skin is made of three layers. Sweat **glands** and oil glands are part of the skin. Sweat glands make sweat. Sweat cools your body when it gets too hot. Oil glands make oil. This oil keeps your skin soft, smooth, and waterproof.

Many teen-agers have a skin problem called **acne**. Adults can have acne, too. People with acne have blackheads, whiteheads, and pimples. People can have acne on the face, back, shoulders, or chest.

What causes acne? During the teen years, oil glands often make too much oil. This oil can block the skin's **pores**. At times the oil in the pores forms whiteheads. Whiteheads look like bumps under the skin. Blackheads form when the oil in blocked pores turns a dark color. Pimples form when blocked pores become **infected**.

How can you care for acne? Bathe every day. Wash your face twice a day using warm water and a gentle soap. Don't scrub your face. Never squeeze blackheads or pimples. This can spread acne. Keep your hair clean. Try not to use make-up, or use only oil-free make-up. Eat a balanced diet. Even with good care, acne can get worse. Your family doctor or a skin doctor can give you medicine to help clear up acne.

Glands are inside your body. Some glands make sweat or oil.

A person has **acne** when tiny openings in the skin become blocked with oil.

Your **pores** are tiny openings in the skin. Oil and sweat come out of your pores.

An area of the body becomes **infected** when bacteria or other germs attack and grow there.

Your skin is made of three layers.

A **fungus** is a very tiny, nongreen plant that sometimes causes disease.

Black or brown spots on the skin are **moles**.

A **sunscreen lotion** blocks the sun's harmful rays from damaging your skin.

SPF stands for sun protection factor. An SPF number tells how much protection a sunscreen provides.

Athlete's foot is caused by a **fungus**. The fungus causes red, cracked, itchy skin between the toes. To prevent athlete's foot, keep your feet dry. Change your socks every day. Try to wear cotton or wool socks. A doctor should treat bad cases of athlete's foot.

Moles can be flat spots or raised bumps. Most moles are not a problem. But some moles do become dangerous cancers. See a doctor if you have a mole that starts to grow or change in size, shape, or color. Go to a doctor right away if a mole bleeds or hurts.

Sunburn is a problem caused by too much time in the sun. The sun's rays can damage your skin. The sun is most harmful to light-colored skin, but it also harms darker skin. The sun can cause skin cancers. It can also make your skin wrinkle at an early age.

Protect your skin from the sun. Always wear **sunscreen lotion** when you are outdoors. Buy a lotion that has **SPF** 15 or a higher number on the label. Put lotion on 30 minutes before you go outside.

At the pool or beach, wear sunscreen lotion and a hat. Put on more lotion after you swim. Use more lotion if you have been sweating a lot, too.

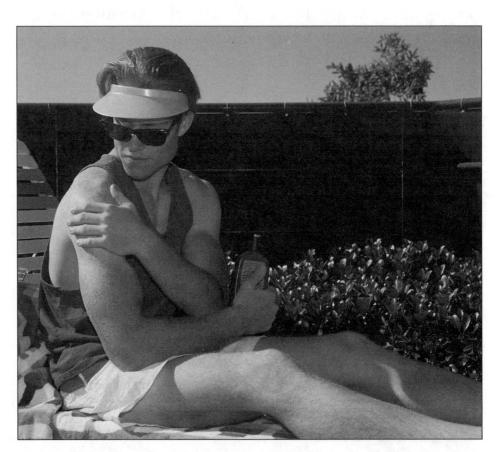

The sun damages skin. Wear sunscreen lotion and a hat to protect yourself outdoors.

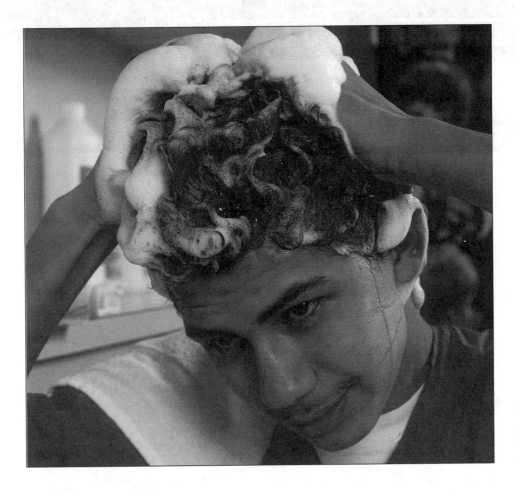

To look your best, wash your hair as often as necessary so it will always look clean.

Your Hair and Nails

Your scalp is the skin that holds your hair on to your head. If the scalp's oil glands make too much oil, you have oily hair. Hair that is not oily can be washed two or three times a week. Oily hair needs to be washed more often. Care for your hair by keeping it clean.

If you have **dandruff**, wash your hair with a dandruff shampoo. If the shampoo does not control your dandruff, you should go to a skin doctor.

Most colds are caused by germs that are on unwashed hands. Wash your hands after using the bathroom. Be sure to wash your hands before eating. Always use warm water and soap when you wash.

Clean your nails by using soap and a small nail brush. Cut or file your fingernails before they grow too long. Cut your toenails straight across.

Your hair, nails, and skin need care each day. By caring for them, you will also be taking care of your physical, social, and emotional health.

Small flakes of dead skin from your scalp are **dandruff**.

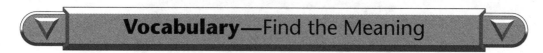

Using What You Learned

Vocabulary—Find the Meaning

Write on your paper the word or words that best complete each sentence.

1. Pimples, blackheads, and whiteheads are _____ .

   acne   **temperature**   **SPF**

2. When you are outdoors, you can protect your skin from the sun's harmful rays by wearing a hat and using a _____ .

   gentle soap   **sunscreen lotion**   **dandruff shampoo**

3. The skin covering your body protects you by keeping your body at the right temperature and keeping out _____ .

   bacteria   **sweat**   **cancer**

4. Black or brown spots on the skin that are either flat or raised are _____ .

   lotion   **moles**   **outdoors**

Comprehension—Write the Questions

Below are the answers for some questions from this chapter. Read each answer. Then write on your paper a possible question to go with each answer. Use the question words to help you.

1. What _____ ?

   Your skin protects your body and keeps it at the right temperature.

2. When _____ ?

   See a doctor if a mole starts to grow or change in size, shape, or color.

3. Where _____ ?

   People get acne on the face, back, shoulders, and chest.

4. How _____ ?

You can prevent athlete's foot by keeping your feet dry and changing your socks every day.

5. What _____ ?

Moles look like brown or black spots on the skin.

6. How _____ ?

Hair that is not oily can be washed two or three times a week.

7. Who _____ ?

The sun is most harmful to people with light-colored skin, but it also harms people with darker skin.

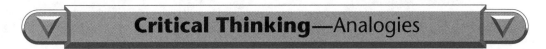

Critical Thinking—Analogies

Use a word or words in the box to finish each sentence. Write the correct answers on your paper.

oil	acne
skin	athlete's foot
shampoo	sun

1. Bicycle helmet is to head as _____ is to body.

2. Soap is to skin as _____ is to hair.

3. Sweat is to body temperature as _____ is to soft skin.

4. Fungus is to athlete's foot as _____ is to skin cancers.

5. Sun is to sunburn as blocked pores are to _____ .

6. Brown spots are to moles as itchy skin is to _____ .

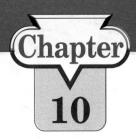

Chapter 10

Caring for Your Teeth

Think About as You Read

- How does plaque cause tooth decay?
- How can you prevent gum disease?
- Why should you avoid eating sugar?

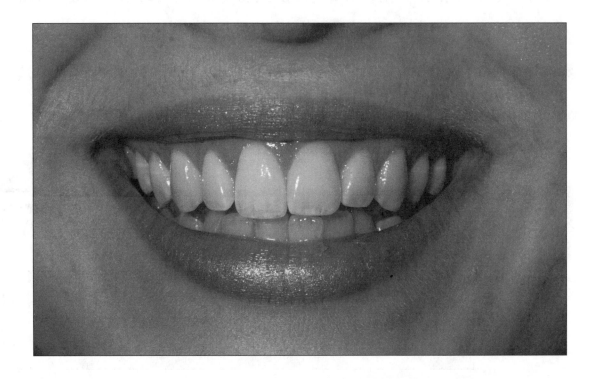

Healthy teeth help you have good health. They help you look your best.

Who is your favorite actor or actress? This person probably has a beautiful smile and healthy teeth. You need healthy teeth to have good health.

Tooth Decay and Gum Disease

Your teeth have a hard, white covering called **enamel**.

Your teeth are made of a very hard material. The part of your teeth that you can see is covered by smooth **enamel**. Each tooth is filled with nerves and blood. A long root holds each tooth in the jawbone. Gums surround the roots.

Bacteria are inside your mouth at all times. These bacteria are always forming **plaque** on your teeth. Plaque can cause tooth decay and gum disease.

Plaque mixes with sugar and starch, which come from food in your mouth, to form acids. These acids can make holes in the tooth enamel. If this decay is not treated, it destroys the tooth. Decay can go down to the root of the tooth. It can cause a toothache. If the tooth cannot be fixed, it must be pulled.

A dentist should always repair teeth that have decay. The dentist may use a drill to clean out the tooth decay. The drill makes a hole around the decay. Then the dentist fills up the hole. The material used to fill the hole is called a filling.

Plaque also causes gum disease. Plaque often forms hard **tartar** on the teeth. Tartar can get under the gums. At first, tartar causes gums to bleed. As more tartar forms under the gums, the gums may become infected. The bones that hold the teeth in the mouth become weak. As the bones weaken, the teeth become loose. Sometimes teeth fall out.

You must go to a dentist if you have gum disease. The dentist removes the tartar so the gums can heal.

Bacteria make a sticky covering called **plaque** on teeth.

The hard material that is caused by plaque and forms on the teeth near the gums is **tartar**.

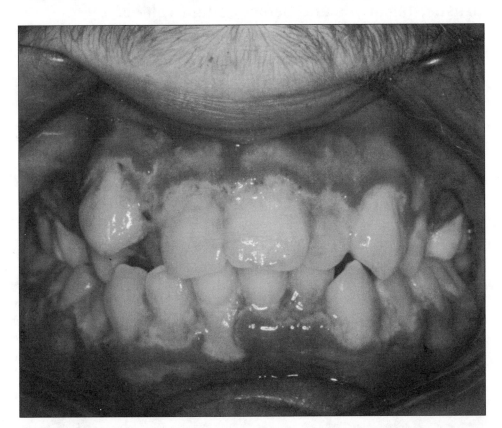

Plaque can cause tooth decay. It can also cause gum disease.

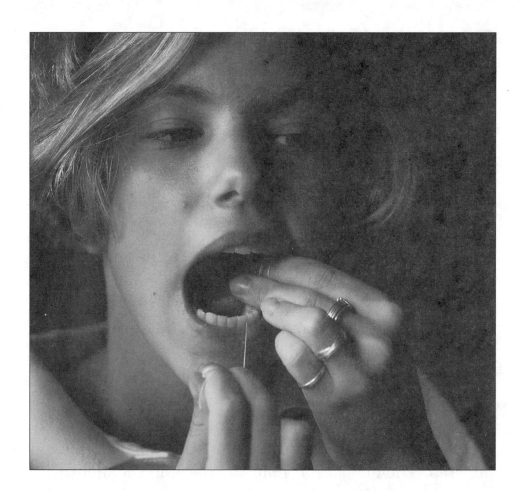

Use dental floss every day. Floss to remove food and plaque from between the teeth.

Preventing Tooth Decay and Gum Disease

Follow these eight rules to have healthy teeth.

1. Brush your teeth at least twice a day. Try to brush after meals and before going to sleep.

2. Brush your teeth correctly. Use a soft, small toothbrush. Hold the brush so it is slanted against your gums. Brush back and forth. Use short, gentle strokes. Brush the tops and sides of your teeth.

3. **Floss** at least once each day. Flossing removes food and plaque from between your teeth. Use both hands to pull the dental floss between all of your teeth. Floss gently under the edge of your gums and around each tooth.

4. Rinse your mouth with water when you cannot brush after eating.

5. Use a **fluoride** toothpaste or mouthwash. Fluoride makes tooth enamel stronger.

6. Eat fewer foods with sugar. Sugar helps form acids that cause decay.

You **floss** when you clean between your teeth, using a strong waxed or unwaxed thread called dental floss.

A chemical that protects teeth from decay is **fluoride**.

7. Eat foods with vitamins C and D and calcium. These nutrients build healthy teeth and gums. Milk, oranges, and vegetables contain these nutrients.

8. Visit a dentist every six months. The dentist will check and clean your teeth.

Malocclusion

A person has a **malocclusion** when the teeth are crowded or crooked in the mouth. Sometimes there are wide spaces between teeth. Sometimes the teeth don't fit together well when biting and chewing.

Malocclusions make teeth less attractive. They can lower a person's self-esteem. Malocclusions make it easier to get tooth decay and gum disease, too.

Orthodontists sometimes put **braces** on people who have malocclusions. Braces gently push the teeth into the correct place in the mouth. It takes about two years to correct a malocclusion.

To have a beautiful smile, you must take good care of your teeth. Healthy teeth can help you look and feel your best.

Orthodontists are dentists who are trained to correct malocclusions.

The wires and bands that are used to move and straighten teeth are **braces**.

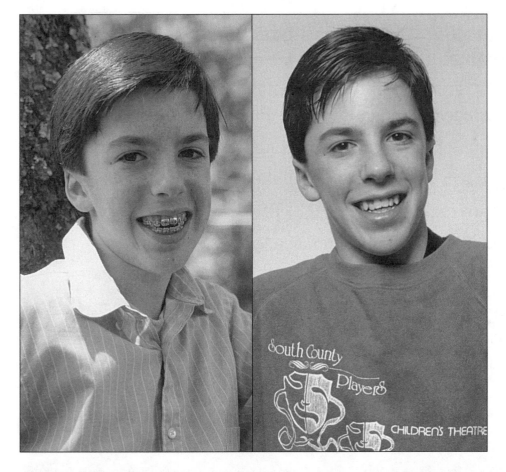

Braces are often used to treat malocclusions. After treatment teeth look more attractive.

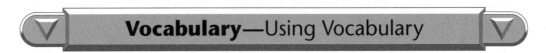

Using What You Learned

Vocabulary—Using Vocabulary

Use each word to write a complete sentence on your paper about dental care.

1. orthodontist
2. enamel
3. floss
4. plaque
5. malocclusion
6. tartar

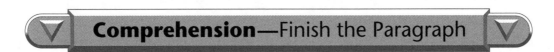

Comprehension—Finish the Paragraph

Number your paper from 1 to 10. Use a word from the box to finish each sentence. Write the correct answers on your paper.

fluoride	starch	teeth	bacteria	dentist
floss	enamel	disease	bleed	calcium

Plaque can cause tooth decay and gum __(1)__ . Plaque is a layer of __(2)__ that forms on your teeth. Plaque forms acids when it mixes with the sugar and __(3)__ from the foods you eat. These acids can make holes in the tooth __(4)__ . Plaque can also form hard tartar on the __(5)__ . Tartar can cause your gums to __(6)__ and become infected. A __(7)__ must remove the tartar so the gums can heal.

To care for your teeth, you should brush and __(8)__ every day. Use a __(9)__ toothpaste to make tooth enamel stronger. Eat foods with vitamins C and D and __(10)__ to help build healthy teeth and gums.

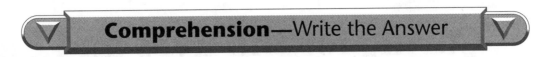

Comprehension—Write the Answer

Write a sentence on your paper to answer each question.

1. What causes the bones in the mouth to become weak and the teeth to become loose?

2. What happens if tooth decay is not treated?

3. How does a dentist repair teeth that have decay?

4. Why is flossing once a day important for keeping your teeth healthy?

5. What kinds of foods are good to eat to build healthy teeth and gums?

6. How do braces help fix malocclusions?

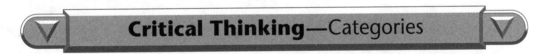

Critical Thinking—Categories

Read the words in each group. Decide how they are alike. Find the best title in the box for each group. Write the title on your paper.

Tartar	Dentist	Dental Care
Enamel	Tooth	Malocclusion

1. enamel
   nerves
   root

2. bleeding gums
   infection
   loose teeth

3. cover
   smooth
   hard

4. brush
   floss
   use fluoride

5. crowded
   orthodontist
   braces

6. drill
   repair
   checkup

Caring for the Eyes and Ears

Think About as You Read

- **How should you take care of your eyes and ears?**
- **What causes an ear infection?**
- **What causes hearing loss?**

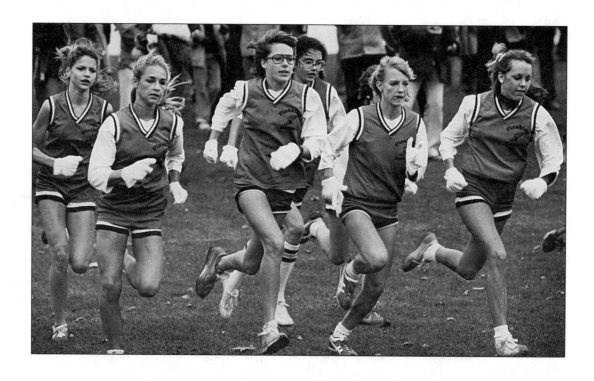

Your eyes and ears help you enjoy many kinds of activities.

You learn many things about the world around you by using your eyes and ears. You use them to enjoy TV and movies. You need to take care of your eyes and ears to keep them healthy.

Common Eye Problems

People with healthy eyes can have vision problems. Many people are **nearsighted**. They cannot clearly see things that are far away. They can only see things that are close to them. Other people are **farsighted**. They cannot clearly see things that are close to them. But they can see things that are far away. An **astigmatism** causes blurred vision. Eyeglasses and contact lenses can correct all three problems.

Another eye problem is **conjunctivitis**. It is very **contagious**. Conjunctivitis can spread from one eye to the other. An infected person can spread conjunctivitis to other people. This happens when other people touch an infected person. It also happens when people touch things that an infected person handled. People with conjunctivitis should always wash their hands after touching their eyes. They should use clean towels. They should separate their own used towels from those used by other people. Conjunctivitis must be treated by a doctor.

Glaucoma is caused by too much pressure within the eye. Your eye doctor can treat glaucoma with special eye drops. People who do not get treatment for glaucoma can lose part or all of their vision.

A person has **conjunctivitis** when part of the eye becomes infected, and the eye looks pink or red. The eye may also itch or have a thick liquid running from it.

A **contagious** illness can be spread easily from one person to another.

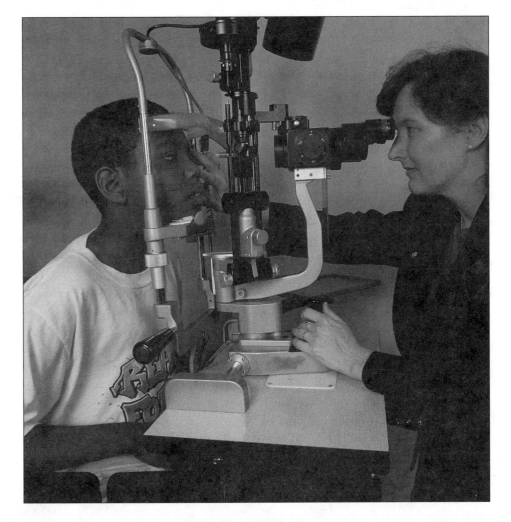

An eye doctor will check for glaucoma during an eye exam.

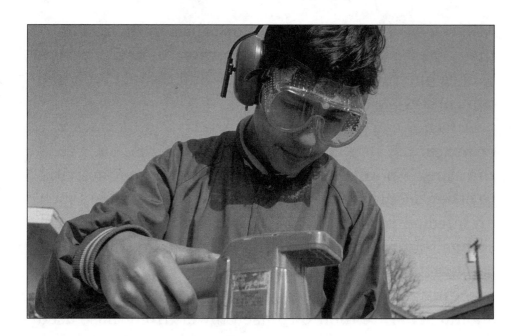

Wear goggles to protect your eyes when you use power tools.

Taking Care of the Eyes

There are six rules to help you protect your eyes.
1. Have an eye exam at least once every two years.
2. Never touch your eyes with dirty hands.
3. Don't share eye make-up. Keep your eye make-up clean.
4. Keep your eyeglasses and contact lenses clean. Wear them as needed.
5. Wear sunglasses when you are in the sun. Buy sunglasses that have a UV protection label. These will protect your eyes from the sun's harmful **ultraviolet rays**.
6. Wear **goggles** when you use power tools. Wear goggles when you play sports.

Goggles are safety glasses that are worn to protect the eyes.

Ear Infections and Hearing Loss

Why do people get ear infections? Cold germs from the nose and throat can travel through the **Eustachian tube** to the ear. Then germs go into a part of the ear called the middle ear. The middle ear becomes infected. An ear infection can cause fever. It can also cause pain in the ear.

Often ear infections must be treated with **antibiotics**. Always see a doctor if the pain in your ear lasts for more than a few hours.

The **Eustachian tube** connects the ear, nose, and throat.

Medicines called **antibiotics** are used to fight diseases caused by bacteria.

Millions of people suffer from hearing loss. This means they have lost some or all of their hearing. Some people are born with a hearing loss. Other people suffer hearing loss from ear infections that are not treated. Hearing loss can also be caused by very loud noises. Listening to very loud music can cause a hearing loss. The more time people spend near loud noises, the greater the hearing loss can be.

A hearing aid can help most people with a hearing loss to hear better. A hearing aid makes sounds louder. It may be worn in or around the ear.

Care of the Ears

These five rules can help you care for your ears.
1. Do not put anything into your ears. Cotton-tipped sticks should not be used to clean your ears.
2. Wear a safety helmet when you play sports.
3. Gently dry your ears after swimming.
4. Gently blow your nose when you have a cold. Try to stop the **mucus** in your nose from going into your ears.
5. Protect your ears from loud noises. Wear special earmuffs that keep out loud noises.

Think of how your eyes and ears help you each day. Take care of them in order to feel good and enjoy life.

Mucus is a sticky liquid that is made by the body. Mucus helps protect the body against germs and dirt.

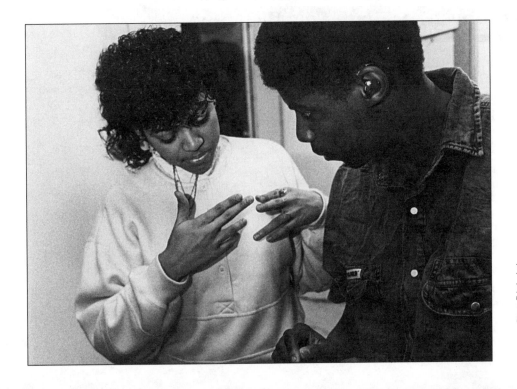

Hearing aids help many people with hearing losses. They help by making sounds louder.

Using What You Learned

Vocabulary—Matching

Match each vocabulary word in **Group B** with a sentence from **Group A** that tells about the word. Write the letter of the correct answer on your paper.

Group A

1. This tube connects your ear, nose, and throat.

2. You can use these safety glasses to protect your eyes.

3. This vision problem causes objects to look blurred.

4. Your doctor may give you these medicines to treat ear infections.

5. This is a contagious eye problem.

6. This sticky liquid helps protect the body against germs and dirt.

Group B

a. astigmatism

b. goggles

c. antibiotics

d. Eustachian

e. mucus

f. conjunctivitis

Comprehension—Write the Answer

Write a sentence on your paper to answer each question.

1. What should people with conjunctivitis do after touching their eyes?

2. How often should you have an eye exam?

3. What are two causes of hearing loss?

4. How should you blow your nose when you have a cold?

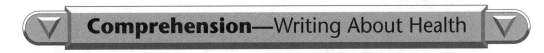

Comprehension—Writing About Health

Answer the following question in complete sentences on your paper.

What can you do to take care of your eyes and ears?

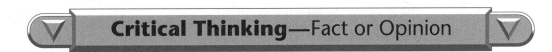

Critical Thinking—Fact or Opinion

Write **Fact** on your paper for each fact below. Write **Opinion** for each opinion. You should find three sentences that are opinions.

1. People with healthy eyes can have problems with their vision.
2. It is better to be nearsighted than it is to be farsighted.
3. Sunglasses that have a UV protection label can be worn to protect your eyes from the sun's ultraviolet rays.
4. Eyeglasses and contact lenses are used to correct an astigmatism.
5. Some people get ear infections because cold germs from the nose and throat go through the Eustachian tube to the ear.
6. A hearing aid can help someone with a hearing loss by making sounds louder.
7. It is easier to take care of your eyes than it is to take care of your ears.
8. A safety helmet can be used to protect your ears when you play sports.
9. It is more important to wear goggles to protect your eyes when you play sports than when you use power tools.
10. Ear infections are often treated with antibiotics.

Chapter 12

Planning Your Personal Health Program

Think About as You Read

- **Why is good posture important?**
- **How can you prevent body odor?**
- **How does sleep help your body?**

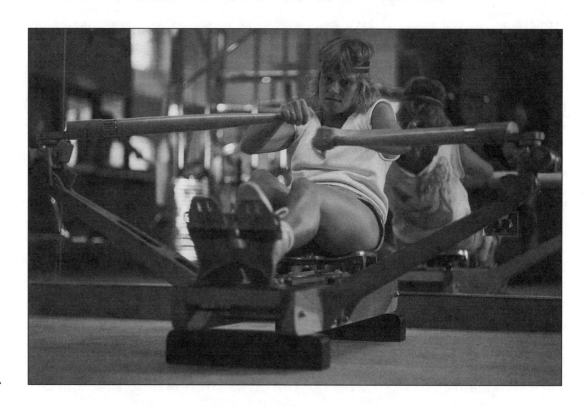

Every person needs a fitness program. Your program should include exercise.

Every person wants a strong, healthy body. Everyone wants healthy eyes, ears, skin, and teeth. You need to plan a health program to reach these health goals.

Planning Your Own Health Program

Your health program must help you in five ways.
1. Plan to have physical fitness by exercising at least three times a week.

2. Take care of your hair, skin, nails, and teeth every day.
3. Do activities you enjoy.
4. Get enough sleep.
5. Have your teeth checked by your dentist every six months. Have your eyes checked by your eye doctor at least once every two years. Visit your family doctor for a checkup once a year.

Your Physical Fitness Plan

Your personal fitness plan should have six steps.
1. Set fitness goals. Decide which fitness skills you want to improve.
2. Choose goals that you can reach. Don't choose goals that are too hard.
3. Choose exercises that help you meet your goal. If your goal is to build the muscles in your arms, do pushups and lift weights.
4. Put your fitness plan into action. As you reach your goals, set new goals.
5. Make time for fitness. Decide the days and times you will exercise.
6. Don't get too tired. A good exercise program should not make you really tired.

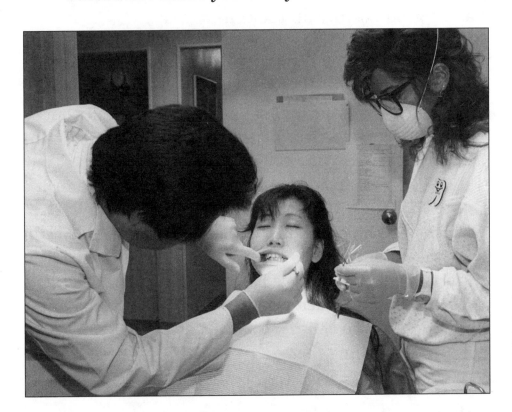

Visit your doctor and dentist for checkups as part of your personal health program.

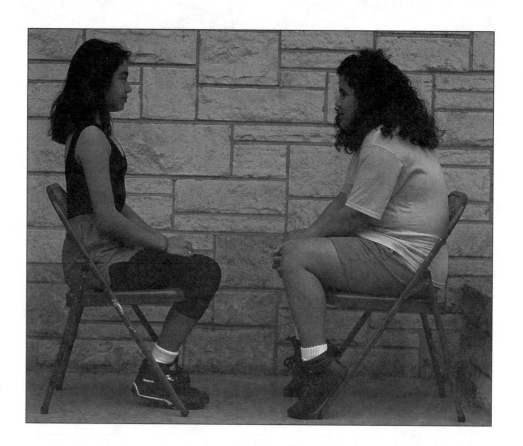

The girl on the left has good sitting posture. The girl on the right has poor posture.

Your physical fitness plan should include exercises for good posture. Good posture helps you look better. It helps raise your self-esteem. When you carry your body correctly, your body parts are in the right places. You can work at making good posture a habit. Think about your posture when you walk, stand, and sit. Practice having good posture all the time.

Grooming

Your personal health program must include time for grooming. Keep your nails and face clean. Wash your hair as often as needed. Brush your teeth at least twice a day. Floss them once a day.

Body odor often becomes a problem during the teen years. People get body odor when their sweat mixes with bacteria that are on their skin. To prevent body odor, take a bath or shower every day. Wash with warm water and soap to remove bacteria that cause body odor. Always wear clean clothes. Body odor sticks to dirty clothes. You can remove the odor from your clothes by washing them.

Many people use **deodorant** to prevent body odor. But a deodorant never takes the place of a bath or shower.

We all have special days and meetings in our lives. Take extra care with your grooming on those days.

A **deodorant** is used to stop body odor by killing bacteria on the skin.

Sleep

Your health program must allow you to get enough sleep. Most teen-agers need nine to ten hours of sleep a night. Sleep gives your body time to rest. Then it can repair itself. Your heart slows down and does less work. You breathe more slowly. Your body does most of its growing while you are sleeping.

Sometimes it is difficult to fall asleep. Here are five ways you can help yourself fall asleep.

1. Listen to soft music that is played quietly.
2. Go to bed about the same time each night.
3. Drink a glass of milk before going to bed.
4. Do something to relax, such as reading.
5. Avoid eating and drinking caffeine. Caffeine is found in coffee, tea, many sodas, and chocolate.

Your health program can help you reach wellness. Allow time for physical fitness, grooming, and sleep in order to look and feel your best each day.

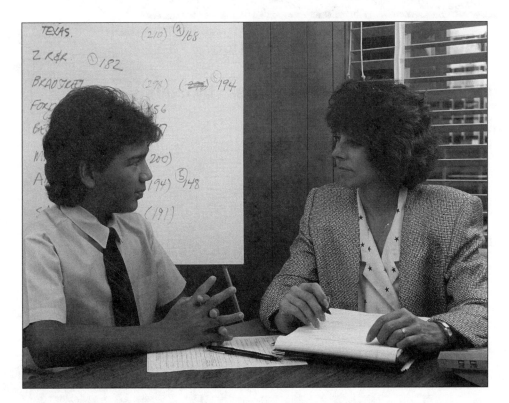

This teen took care of his grooming before he went for this summer job interview.

Using What You Learned

Vocabulary—Finish the Sentence

Choose a word or words from the box to complete each sentence. Write the correct answers on your paper.

repair	bacteria	deodorant
checkup	posture	physical fitness

1. Try to have good _____ when you walk, stand, and sit.

2. You can help prevent body odor by using a _____ .

3. You improve your _____ when you exercise at least three times a week.

4. Deodorant kills _____ that cause odor.

5. Sleep gives your body time to rest and _____ itself.

6. Visit your family doctor for a _____ once a year.

Comprehension—Write the Answer

Write a sentence on your paper to answer each question.

1. How often should you plan to have physical fitness by exercising?

2. Why is it important to have good posture?

3. When does your body do most of its growing?

4. How often should you brush and floss your teeth?

5. How does deodorant help prevent body odor?

6. How many hours of sleep do most teen-agers need?

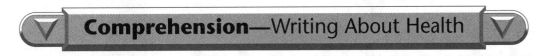

Comprehension—Writing About Health

Answer the following question in complete sentences on your paper.

What kinds of physical activity do you do every week?

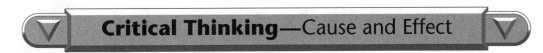

Critical Thinking—Cause and Effect

Write sentences on your paper by matching each cause on the left with an effect on the right.

Cause

1. You want to have good physical fitness, so _____

2. You want to help yourself fall asleep, so _____

3. You have set a goal to build the muscles in your legs, so _____

4. You want to remove the body odor from your dirty clothes, so _____

5. You eat and drink too much caffeine, so _____

6. You have reached your physical fitness goals, so _____

7. You want to make good posture a habit, so _____

Effect

a. you have trouble falling asleep.

b. you wash your dirty clothes.

c. you set new goals.

d. you exercise three times a week and eat a balanced diet.

e. you listen to soft music that is played quietly.

f. you think about your posture when you walk, stand, and sit.

g. you have started doing leg exercises to meet that goal.

UNIT 5

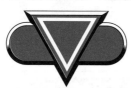

Safety and First Aid

Do you know what to do when there is an emergency? Imagine you are at a friend's house. Your friend's father burns his hand while cooking. Would you know how to help him? Knowing what to do when there is an emergency can help you reach your goal of wellness.

To enjoy life you need to be safe at home and away from home. By learning about safety, you can protect yourself from danger. By learning how to give first aid, you will be able to help someone who is hurt.

Have You Ever Wondered?

▼ Sometimes people are attacked while walking down the street. How can you protect yourself?

▼ Most accidents happen at home. How can you make your home a safer place?

▼ You must call for help in an emergency. Whom should you call, and what should you say?

As you read this unit, think about how you can protect your health. Learning about safety and first aid will help you have wellness.

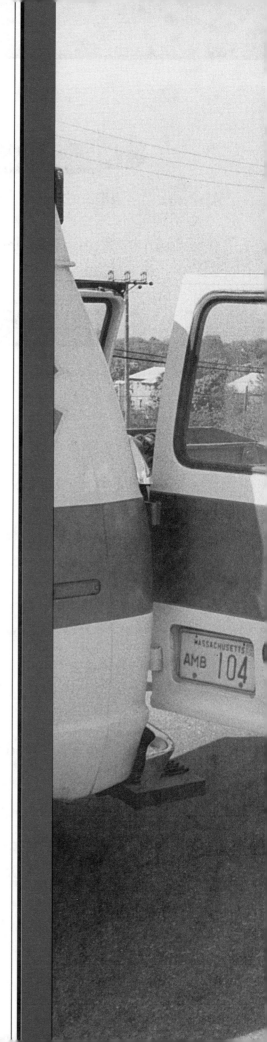

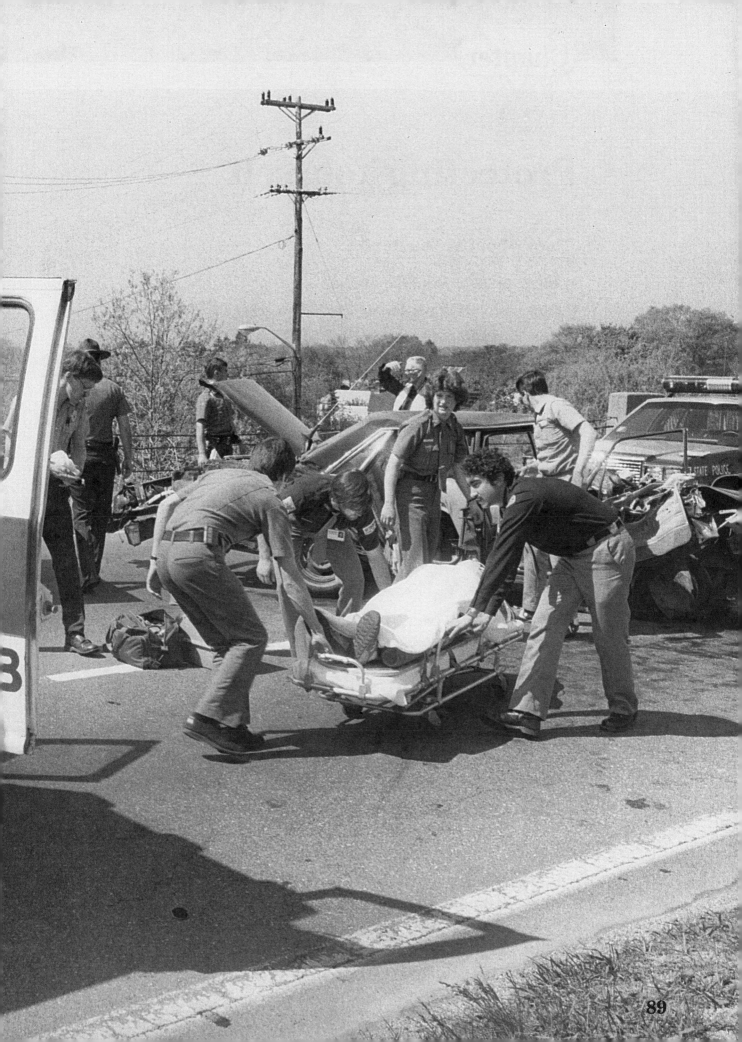

Chapter 13

Protecting Yourself

Think About as You Read

- What are four kinds of abuse?
- How can young people protect themselves from abuse?
- How can you protect yourself from violent crime?

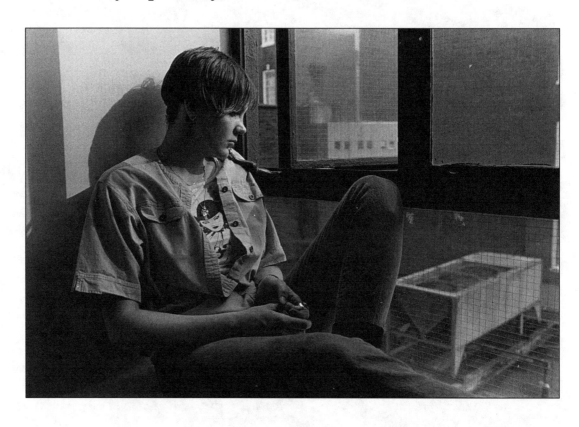

Many young people are abused. They may not be given enough food, clothing, and care.

Carlos is worried about Kim, a girl who goes to his school. Kim always looks sad and tired. Her hair, face, and clothes are always dirty. She wears only a thin jacket on very cold, wet days. Carlos decides to tell his teacher about Kim. Carlos believes his teacher can help Kim or get her some help.

Each year many young people are hurt by adults. The adult may even be a parent. Learning how to protect yourself is an important part of wellness.

Understanding Abuse

Abuse means hurting someone in a way that is not an accident. You should protect yourself from four types of abuse.

1. **Neglect** is the type of abuse that happens most often. The young person who is neglected does not receive enough care. The young person may not be given enough food and clean clothing. The young person may not be taken to a doctor even when he or she is very sick.

2. Physical abuse hurts the body. The young person may be beaten, pushed, or burned. Physical abuse can cause bruises, cuts, and broken bones.

3. Emotional abuse happens when people always yell at, **criticize**, or say things to hurt the young person. This lowers the young person's self-esteem.

To **criticize** is to find something wrong with what a person does or says.

4. Sexual abuse happens when an adult behaves in a sexual way towards a young person. Sexual abuse is often done by a family member.

Abused young people may seem very sad. They may avoid spending time with friends. They may have cuts and other bruises from being pushed and hit. Abused young people have very low self-esteem. Some may talk about killing themselves.

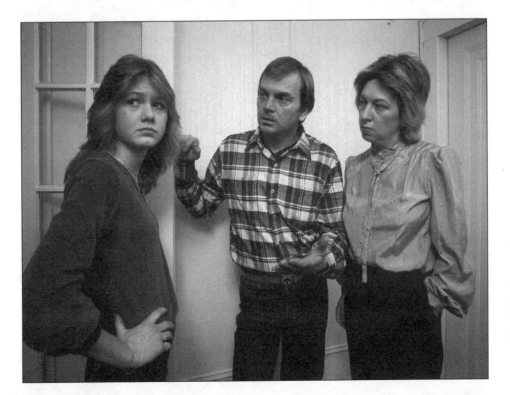

This teen has been emotionally abused many times. Abuse has lowered her self-esteem.

Abusers come from every race and religion. They can be rich or poor. Abusers may often use drugs or alcohol. They are often teen-age parents. Most people who abuse others were abused when they were children.

You have the right to be safe. Work on building your own self-esteem. Then you will find it easier to stop people from abusing you. Use these five rules to protect yourself from abuse.

1. Trust your feelings. If you feel that you are being abused, you are probably correct.
2. Don't keep abuse a secret. Tell an adult whom you trust.
3. Avoid being alone with people who do or say things that make you feel **uncomfortable**. Also avoid being alone with people you do not know or trust.
4. When abuse begins, tell the abuser to stop the unwanted behavior.
5. Remove yourself from the problem.

The Danger of Violent Crimes

Many people are **victims** of **violent** crimes. **Homicide** and **rape** are violent crimes.

You are **uncomfortable** when someone does or says things that make you feel afraid.

Victims are people who are harmed or killed by another person.

To be **violent** means to act with strong force.

The killing of one person by another person is a **homicide**.

Rape is a crime where force is used by an attacker to perform sexual acts on another person.

You have the right to be safe. Avoid being alone with people you do not know or trust.

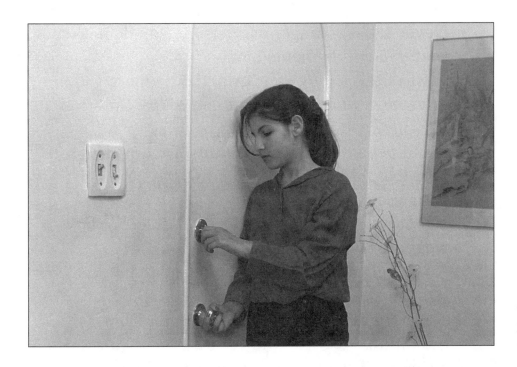

Keep your house doors and windows locked to protect yourself from violent crimes.

What causes one person to kill another? People who use alcohol or drugs sometimes lose control of themselves. Sometimes these people become so angry during an argument that they kill a person.

Males and females both can be raped. During a rape the attacker uses force to perform sexual acts on another person. Most victims of rape are raped by someone they know.

What should you do if you are raped? Report the crime to the police at once. The police will have a doctor check your body for proof that you were raped. So do not bathe or shower until the police have the proof they need. This proof will be used in court against the person who raped you.

Rape can lower a victim's self-esteem. So rape victims always need emotional help.

You can protect yourself against violent crimes. Here are some rules to follow.

1. Be careful. Avoid walking alone.
2. Do not talk about your jewelry or money.
3. Keep your house doors and windows locked.
4. Do not let strangers into your home. Use a peephole or look out of a window to see who is outside your door.

A **guardian** is an adult who is responsible for taking care of the needs of a young person.

5. Never tell a stranger or someone you do not trust that you will be home alone.
6. Always tell a parent or **guardian** where you are going and when you plan to be home. Call that person if you know you will be late.
7. Avoid people who are drinking or using drugs.
8. Leave a place quickly if you feel you are in danger.
9. If a person tries to harm you but does not have a weapon, try to run away.
10. Avoid being alone with people you do not know or trust.
11. Never go anywhere with a stranger. Do not hitchhike.

Monica and Jill knew how to be safe. They stayed together while they shopped at the mall. Then they waited together for a bus. A car stopped at the curb by the girls. The driver asked them if they wanted a ride. Monica and Jill said no because they did not want to ride with a stranger. But the driver would not leave. The girls felt they might be in danger. So they went back into the mall to get help.

Protecting your safety should be one of your goals. You have the right to be safe at all times.

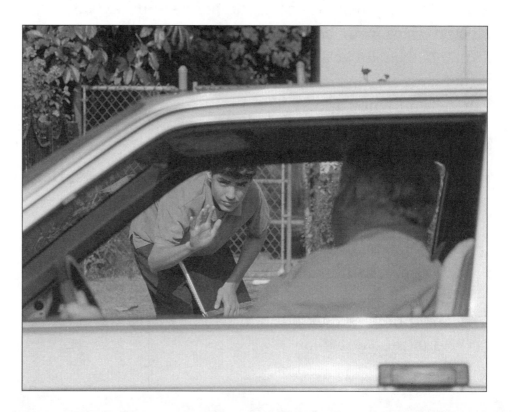

Never accept car rides from strangers.

94

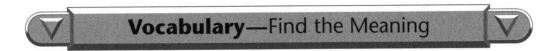

Using What You Learned

Write on your paper the word that best completes each sentence.

1. Hurting someone in a way that is not an accident is _____ .

   proof   **abuse**   **self-esteem**

2. _____ is a crime in which an attacker performs sexual acts on another person by using force.

   Rape   **Neglect**   **Homicide**

3. A person who is hurt by a violent crime is a _____ .

   stranger   **guardian**   **victim**

4. Someone makes you _____ by saying things that make you afraid.

   uncomfortable   **violent**   **criticize**

5. You should call your parent or _____ if you know you will be late getting home.

   stranger   **guardian**   **victim**

Write **True** on your paper for each sentence that is true. Write **False** on your paper for each sentence that is false. There are three false sentences. Rewrite the false sentences on your paper to make them true.

1. Emotional abuse happens when someone hurts your body.

2. Homicide is a violent crime in which one person kills another.

3. Most people who abuse others were once abused themselves.

4. It is safe to get into a car with a friendly stranger.

5. Learning to protect yourself from abuse is an important part of wellness.

6. The type of abuse that happens most often is neglect.

7. A person who is physically abused can get bruises, cuts, and broken bones.

8. Abused people usually have high self-esteem.

9. Drugs or alcohol may be used by abusers.

10. If you feel you are being abused, you should tell an adult whom you trust.

Critical Thinking—Drawing Conclusions

Read the paragraph. Then use the six steps below to decide what to do about someone who makes you feel uncomfortable. Write complete sentences on your paper to answer each question.

Imagine that your parents are having your aunts, uncles, and cousins over for dinner. You used to enjoy seeing all of them. But lately one of the adult relatives has been doing and saying things that make you feel uncomfortable. This person always wants to hug and kiss you when you are alone in a room.

Step 1. What is the problem?

Step 2. What are two ways to solve the problem?

Step 3. What is one consequence for each choice listed in Step 2?

Step 4. Which choice do you think is best?

Step 5. What can you do to put your decision into action?

Step 6. Think about your decision. Why was this the best choice for you?

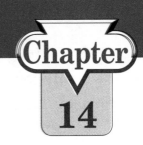

Safety at Home and Away from Home

Think About as You Read

- How can you prevent accidents from happening at home?
- How can car accidents be prevented?
- How can you be safe outdoors?

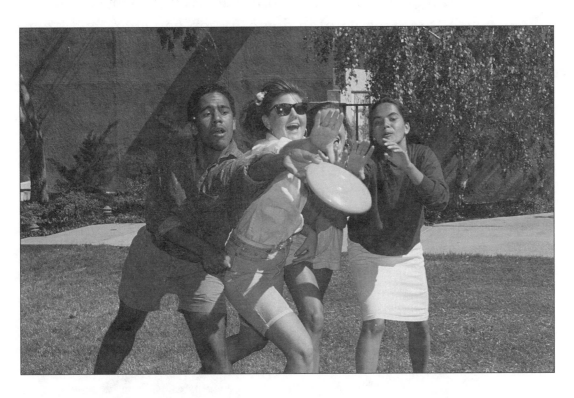

People have more fun when they do not get hurt. Learn to be safe at home and outdoors.

Imagine going to the park for a picnic with friends. To have a good time, everyone must be safe. Learning how to prevent accidents at home and away from home helps you stay safe.

Preventing Falls and Kitchen Accidents

Many falls happen in homes. Try to prevent people from slipping on your floors. Always wipe spills from the floor. Do not leave toys or other objects where people can fall on them.

97

Many people fall on stairs. Stairs should never be slippery. They should not have loose carpeting. A stairway should always be well lit. There should be a light by the top step and the bottom step. A stairway needs to have a handrail. You should hold on to the handrail when walking on the stairs.

Many falls happen in the bathroom. To prevent these falls, use a rubber bath mat in the tub and shower.

Many people fall when they reach for things that are in high places. To reach for these things safely, stand on a strong ladder. Always open the ladder completely. Do not stand on the top step of the ladder.

Many accidents happen in the kitchen. Carry knives with their tips pointed down. When you chop food, turn the tip of the knife away from your body.

Use mixers, blenders, **food processors**, and **garbage disposals** safely. Turn these machines off and wait for the blades to stop moving before you handle them.

Learn to use your oven and stove safely. Do not allow children to play near a hot stove. Always turn the handles of your pots toward the back of the stove. Use pot holders when handling hot pots, pans, and dishes.

Food processors are electric machines that chop, grind, and blend foods.

Garbage disposals in sinks grind food to get rid of it.

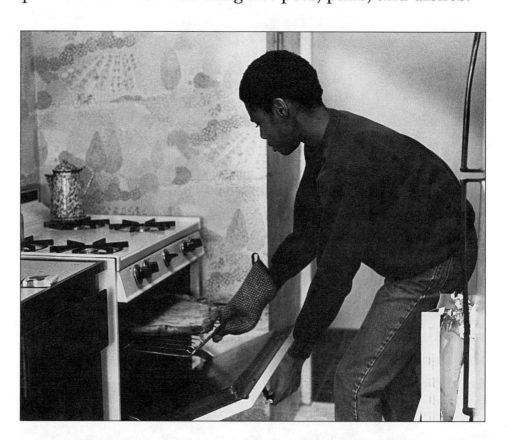

Always use pot holders when handling hot pots, pans, and dishes.

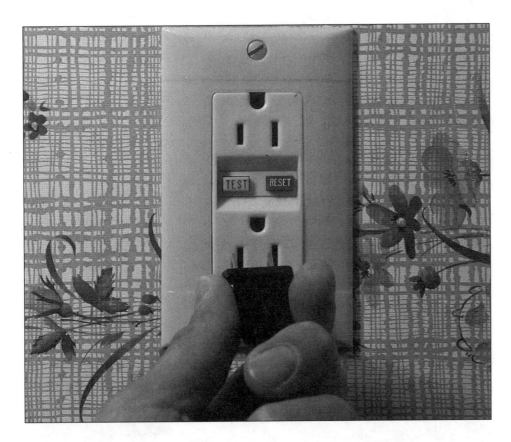

Pull a cord out of an outlet by its plug.

What should you do if a fire starts while food is cooking in the oven? Leave the food in the oven. Turn the oven off. Throw baking soda on the fire. Close the oven door. The fire will go out.

Carefully watch a pan that is on the stove if you are cooking with oil. The oil can catch on fire if it becomes too hot. Never put water on this kind of fire. Put salt or baking soda on it. Cover the pan. Then wait for the fire to go out.

Electrical Accidents and Home Fires

Electric appliances can cause electric shocks. Electric shocks happen when electricity passes through the body. Electric shock can make the body shake or cause burns. To prevent electric shocks, never get appliances wet while you are using them. Be sure your hands are dry when you use a hair dryer.

You can prevent electrical fires. Replace worn-out cords and plugs. Pull cords out of an **outlet** by their plugs. Do not plug too many appliances into one outlet. This can cause a fire.

An **outlet** is a place for plugging in an electric appliance.

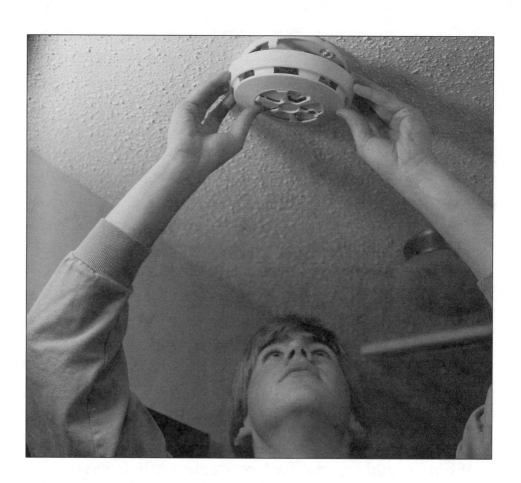

Smoke detectors buzz when there is smoke nearby.

Things that can easily catch on fire are **flammable**.

Every year people die in home fires. Cigarette smoking is the leading cause of home fires. Many fires start when people smoke in bed. Sometimes cigarette ashes fall onto the sheets and blankets. They quickly catch on fire. People should never smoke in bed.

Flammable liquids like paint and gasoline burn easily. Keep these liquids in closed jars or cans. Store them far away from your stove, heater, or water heater.

Smoke detectors can help protect you. They buzz when there is smoke nearby. Every floor of your house needs a smoke detector. Check the batteries once a month to make sure your smoke detectors are working.

Everyone needs a plan for escaping from a home fire. Practice your plan during home fire drills. During a fire there is less smoke near the floor. So crawl on the floor as you leave the house. Decide on a place where people can meet outside the house. After leaving the burning house, one person should call the fire department for help. Never go back into the burning house.

100

Car and Pedestrian Safety

More children, teen-agers, and young adults die from car accidents than from any other cause. To be safe when riding in a car, always wear a seat belt. Wear a **shoulder harness** if it is part of the seat belt.

Drunk drivers cause more than half of all car accidents. Never get into a car with a driver who has been drinking alcohol. It is against the law to drink alcohol and drive a car.

How can you and other **pedestrians** be safe? Always cross streets at corners. Obey traffic signs and traffic lights. It is safer to walk on the sidewalk than in the street. If there is no sidewalk, walk on the left side of the road. Always face the traffic as you walk.

A **shoulder harness** is the part of the seat belt worn across the shoulder. It helps protect a person from being thrown forward during a car accident.

People who walk down the street are **pedestrians**.

Pool and Bicycle Safety

Many people drown each year. Protect yourself by learning how to swim. Follow all the safety rules posted at a pool or beach. Go swimming only if a lifeguard is working by the pool or beach. Never swim in a dark pool or at the beach at night. Never go swimming if you have been drinking alcohol or using drugs. Avoid swimming alone.

Protect yourself from drowning by learning how to swim.

101

To **tread** water is to keep your head above water and the rest of your body straight up and down. Do this with an up-and-down movement of your feet and sometimes your arms.

What should you do if you are drowning? Call for help. Wave your arms to show people that you need help. While you are waiting for help, try to float or **tread** water. Never pretend that you are drowning.

Tell a lifeguard if you see a person drowning. You can throw a life jacket to the person. As you stand on land, try carefully handing a long pole to the person drowning. If the victim grabs the pole, you can pull the person out of the water.

Many people enjoy riding bikes. Always wear a helmet when you ride your bike. Ride a bike that has reflectors on the front and back. Your bike should have a side-view mirror to help you see the traffic that is behind you.

To ride your bike safely, obey all traffic rules. Ride to the right of the cars. Travel in the same direction as the cars. Use hand signals when you make turns or stop. Never wear headphones when riding your bike.

Use safety skills in your home and outdoors. Good safety habits can help you reach your goal of wellness.

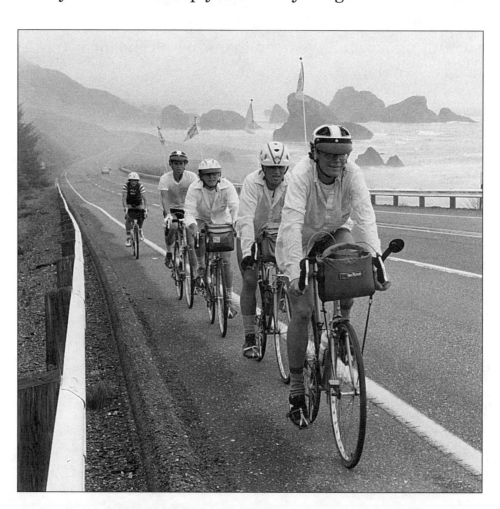

Your bike should have reflectors and a side-view mirror. Wear a helmet when you ride a bike.

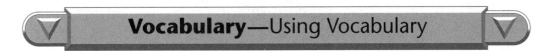

Using What You Learned

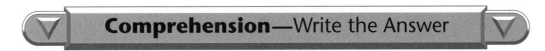

Vocabulary—Using Vocabulary

Use the word or words to write a complete sentence on your paper about safety.

1. outlet
2. smoke detectors
3. pedestrians

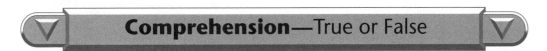

Comprehension—Write the Answer

Write a sentence on your paper to answer each question.

1. What should you do if you spill something on the floor?
2. How can you safely pull an electrical cord from an outlet?
3. Where should flammable liquids be stored?
4. On which side of the street should you walk if there is no sidewalk?
5. Whom should you tell if you see a person drowning?

Comprehension—True or False

Write **True** on your paper for each sentence that is true. Write **False** on your paper for each sentence that is false. There are four false sentences. Rewrite the false sentences on your paper to make them true.

1. To prevent people from falling, you should not leave toys and other objects on the floor.
2. Stairways should have a light at the top and at the bottom for safety.
3. To prevent falls in the bathroom, loose rugs should be in the tub and shower.

103

4. It is safe to stand on chairs and countertops to reach things in high places.

5. When you cut food with a knife, you should turn the tip of the knife away from your body.

6. It is important to turn the handles of your pots toward the front of the stove.

7. If a fire starts in your oven, you should leave the food in it and turn the oven off.

8. An oil fire should be put out with salt or baking soda.

9. It is safer to walk in the street than on the sidewalk.

10. When you ride a bicycle, you should always travel in the same direction as the cars.

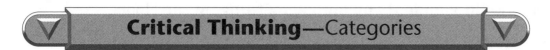

Critical Thinking—Categories

Read the words in each group. Decide how they are alike. Find the best title in the box for each group. Write the title on your paper.

| Causes of Falls | Electrical Safety | Cooking-Oil Fire |
| Pedestrian Safety | Drowning | Bicycle Safety |

1. objects on floors
   poorly lit stairs
   slippery tubs and showers

2. obey traffic rules
   use reflectors on the front and back
   wear a safety helmet

3. replace worn-out cords
   pull plugs from outlets
   keep appliances dry while you use them

4. call for help
   wave your arms
   tread water

5. cross at corners
   obey traffic signs and lights
   walk on sidewalks

6. never use water
   use salt or baking soda
   cover the pan

First Aid

Think About as You Read

- How do you call for emergency help?
- Which accidents always need emergency care?
- How can you help a person who stops breathing?

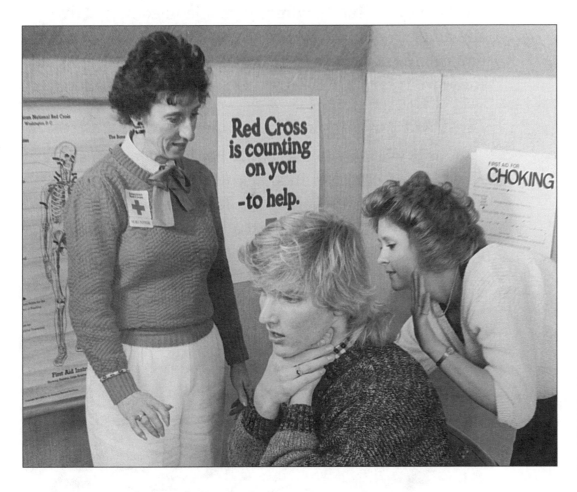

First aid can save a choking person. Would you know how to save another person?

Lydia was in a restaurant when she saw a man choking. She stayed calm and used first aid to help the man. Lydia helped save his life.

First aid is the emergency care given to a hurt or sick person until a doctor can see that person. If you know first aid, you may be able to save a person's life.

Calling for Emergency Help

Most towns or cities have emergency medical services, called EMS. In many places the EMS phone number is 911. If you do not know the phone number for EMS, dial 0. You will speak with a telephone operator. The operator will connect you to EMS.

Keep a list of emergency phone numbers near your phone. This list should have the phone numbers for EMS, the police, and the fire department. It should also list phone numbers for your doctor, the nearest hospital, and the poison control center.

When you call for emergency help, tell what the emergency is. Tell how many people need help. Give the address and phone number of the place where the emergency is. The people you speak to at EMS may ask for more information about the victim or victims.

First Aid for Shock, Wounds, and Animal Bites

People who have been badly hurt can go into shock. An accident victim is in shock when the heartbeat speeds up and blood pressure drops. Shock can cause death. Cover the victim with a blanket to keep that person warm. Call EMS for help right away.

Keep emergency phone numbers near your phone. In an emergency call EMS for help.

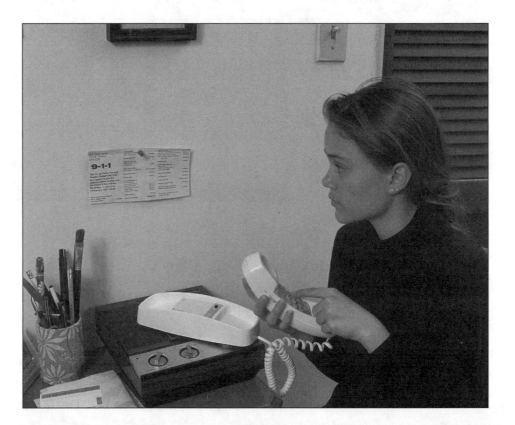

106

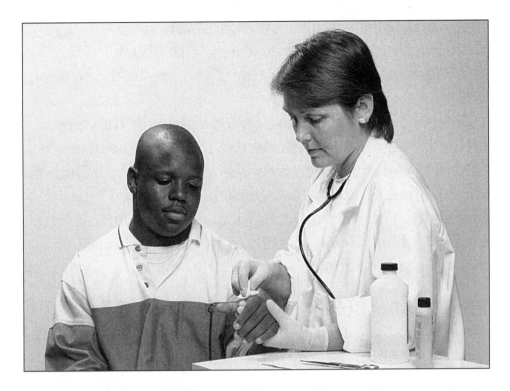

Always wear latex gloves when treating wounds. Throw away used gloves.

Wounds also need first aid. Your skin should never touch another person's blood. Be sure to wear **latex** gloves when treating any kind of wound. Then throw away the used gloves.

Small wounds are small cuts or scratches. Wash these wounds with soap and water. Cover them with **sterile** bandages.

A deep wound can be very dangerous. A deep wound is made when a sharp object makes a hole in the skin. **Tetanus** bacteria may be on a rusty nail or dirty knife that causes a deep wound. The bacteria can cause the person to get a disease called tetanus. People can die from getting tetanus.

Wash a deep wound with soap and water. Cover it with a sterile bandage. A person with a deep wound must see a doctor. The person may need a shot for protection against tetanus.

Some wounds cause a large amount of bleeding. People can die if they lose much blood. So try to slow or stop the flow of blood. Cover the wound with a sterile pad or a clean cloth. Press hard on the wound until the bleeding stops. Be sure to keep the wound covered after the bleeding stops. Call EMS for help.

Wounds are cuts or scratches or bites.

Latex is a material like rubber.

A **sterile** bandage is free from dirt or germs.

Tetanus is a dangerous disease that is caused by a bacteria that enters the body through a wound.

Animal bites are also wounds. Wash animal bites with soap and water. Cover them with sterile bandages. Always see a doctor if you are bitten by an animal.

People can get a disease called **rabies** if they are bitten by an animal with rabies. Rabies can cause death. If you are bitten by someone's pet, try to find out if it has had all its rabies shots. If the animal has not had shots, you may need shots to protect yourself from getting rabies. If you are bitten by a wild animal, you must get rabies shots.

First Aid for Burns and Poisoning

There are three kinds of burns. With a **first-degree burn**, the skin is painful and red. Put cold water on a first-degree burn. Cover it with a sterile bandage.

A **second-degree burn** is very painful. The skin is damaged and may have blisters. Put cold water on the burn. Cover it with a sterile bandage. You must see a doctor.

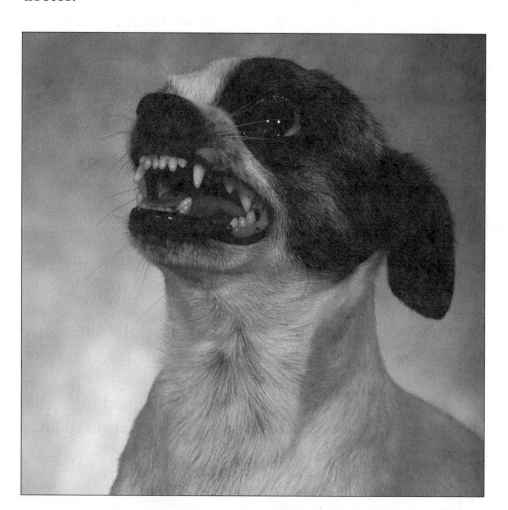

If you are bitten by a dog, try to find out if it has had all of its rabies shots.

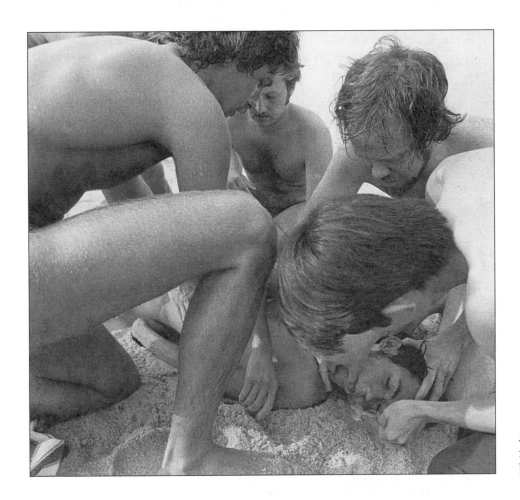

Always check to see if an injured person has stopped breathing.

A **third-degree burn** causes a large amount of damage to every layer of skin. Do not touch a third-degree burn. Carefully cover the burn with a sterile bandage. Call EMS for help.

Work quickly if a person eats or drinks poison. Poison can kill. If the victim is awake, find out which poison was swallowed. Call the poison control center right away. Tell the person at the center which poison the victim swallowed. The person at the center will tell you what to do. Sometimes you cannot find out what kind of poison was swallowed. The victim may be **unconscious**. You must call EMS for help at once.

Helping a Person Who Chokes or Stops Breathing

A person who chokes or stops breathing needs help quickly. Without help that person will soon die. A person who is choking cannot breathe, talk, or cough. People who are choking often grab their throat.

People are **unconscious** when they have passed out, and they cannot feel things or think.

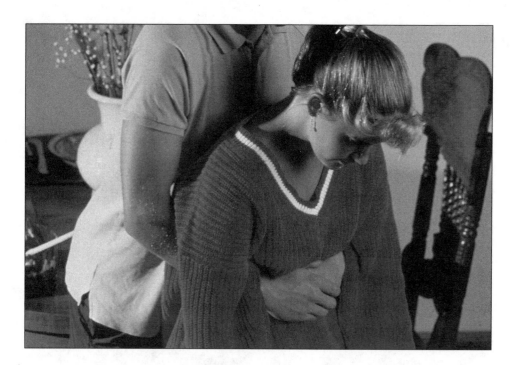

Save a choking person by doing abdominal thrusts.

The **abdomen** is the part of your body that is below your chest and above your hips.

Use the **abdominal thrust** to save a choking person. Have another person call for help.

1. Stand behind the choking person. Put your arms around the person's waist.
2. Make a fist with one hand.
3. Put the thumb of your fist on the person's **abdomen** below the ribs.
4. Push your fist into the abdomen with your other hand. Do quick, hard, upward pushes.
5. Keep doing quick, hard pushes until the person coughs out the object that caused choking.

There are two ways you can help yourself if you are choking. Place the thumb of your fist against your abdomen. Push your fist into your abdomen with your free hand. Do this until you cough up the object. You can also bend forward over the back of a chair. Quickly push your abdomen as hard as you can against the chair. Do this until you cough up the object.

People may stop breathing if they have a heart attack, are in a bad accident, swallow poison, or almost drown. People who suffer electric shock or become unconscious may stop breathing, too. Taking too much alcohol, drugs, or medicine can stop a person's breathing.

Always check to see if an injured person has stopped breathing. When breathing stops, the chest stops moving. No air comes out of the victim's mouth or nose. The victim's lips and fingernails turn blue.

As soon as you know that a person has stopped breathing, start rescue breathing. Follow these steps.

1. Stay calm.
2. Call for emergency help.
3. Lay the victim flat on his or her back.
4. Push the head back. Close the nose with your fingers. Cover the mouth with your mouth.
5. Breathe hard into the victim's mouth. Repeat every five seconds.
6. Do not stop rescue breathing until the person starts to breathe or EMS arrives.

It is important to know what to do in an emergency. One day you may use first aid to help other people.

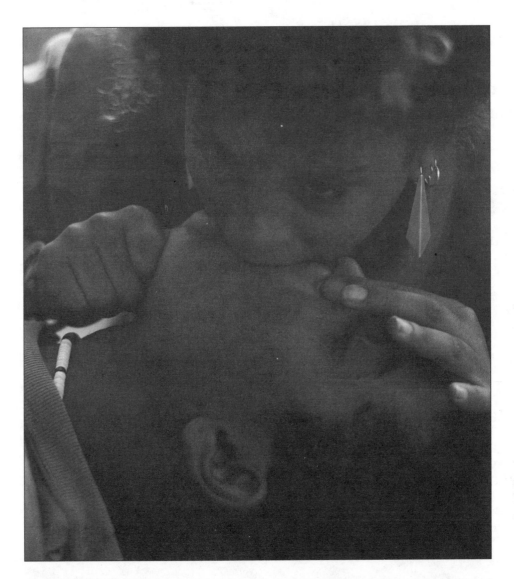

Use rescue breathing to save a person who is not breathing. Ask someone else to call EMS.

Using What You Learned

Vocabulary—Matching

Match each vocabulary word in **Group B** with a sentence from **Group A** that tells about the word. Write the letter of the correct answer on your paper.

Group A

1. These cuts need first aid.

2. This is the most dangerous type of burn.

3. You can use this to save a person who is choking.

4. This describes a person who has passed out.

5. Animals and people can be killed by this disease.

6. This disease can enter a person's body through a wound from a rusty nail.

Group B

a. abdominal thrust

b. unconscious

c. wounds

d. third-degree

e. tetanus

f. rabies

Comprehension—Finish the Paragraph

Number your paper from 1 to 9. Use a word or words from the box to finish each sentence. Write the correct answers on your paper.

sterile	blanket	address
calm	rescue breathing	latex
shock	stopped	operator

It is important to stay __(1)__ in an emergency. Check to see if the person who is sick or hurt has __(2)__ breathing. If the person is not breathing, you should do __(3)__ to save the person.

Some wounds cause a lot of bleeding. Try to stop or slow the flow of blood by covering the wound with a __(4)__ pad or cloth. Wear __(5)__ gloves to keep the blood off your skin.

Remember that a person who is badly hurt can go into __(6)__ . So use a __(7)__ to keep the person warm. Call EMS or the telephone __(8)__ for help. Be sure to give the __(9)__ and the phone number of the place where the emergency is. Explain what the emergency is and answer any questions the people at EMS ask you.

Critical Thinking—Analogies

Use a word from the box to finish each sentence. Write the correct answers on your paper.

blisters	EMS	wound	sterile
shock	poison	tetanus	abdomen

1. Rescue breathing is to mouth as the abdominal thrust is to _____ .

2. EMS is to deep wounds as poison control center is to _____ .

3. First-degree burn is to red skin as second-degree burn is to _____ .

4. Awake is to unconscious as infected is to _____ .

5. Sterile bandages are to wounds as blankets are to _____ .

6. Dialing 0 is to operator as dialing 911 is to _____ .

7. Cold water is to first-degree burn as soap and water are to _____ .

8. Animal bite is to rabies as dirty knife is to _____ .

Safety During Natural Disasters

Think About as You Read

- What supplies do you need at home for emergencies?
- How can you survive earthquakes?
- How can you survive dangerous storms?

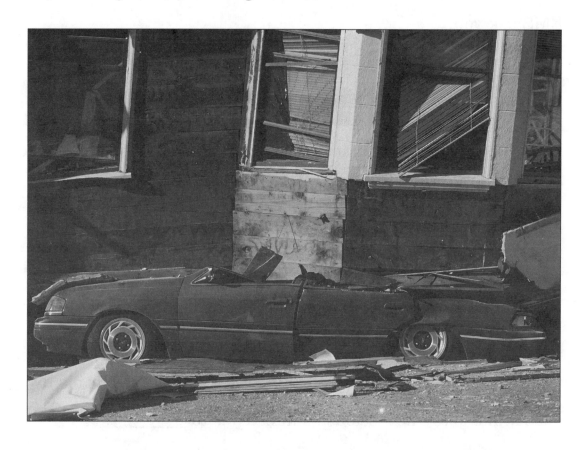

An earthquake damaged this area. Do you know how to be safe during natural disasters?

Imagine being in a room that is shaking during an earthquake. Knowing how to protect yourself during a **natural disaster** is important.

A **natural disaster** is an accident caused by nature.

Being Prepared for Emergencies

We cannot prevent natural disasters. But we should keep supplies in our homes for such emergencies. During natural disasters many homes do not have electricity or running water. So always have bottled water and a radio that runs on batteries. You need at least one flashlight in your home. Have plenty of new batteries for the radio and the flashlight. You should also have candles and matches. You will need blankets and a first-aid kit. You should have a supply of canned food, too.

Listen to weather reports on the radio and TV. They will warn about possible hurricanes or tornadoes. Snowstorms and lightning storms are also reported.

Surviving Earthquakes

During earthquakes the ground shakes and cracks. Earthquakes often last less than a minute. But there can be a large amount of damage. Buildings, bridges, and highways can fall down. Telephone and electric power lines can fall down, too. Water and natural-gas lines can break.

You can **survive** an earthquake. If you are indoors, try to stay in a doorway between two rooms. You can also sit under a strong desk or table. Stay away from windows because you may be hit by broken glass. Do not touch electric lines that have fallen. They can shock you or cause fires.

To **survive** means to go on living even though there are problems.

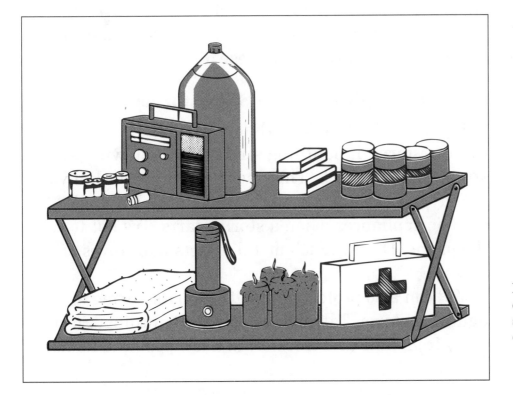

Be prepared for emergencies. Always keep supplies in your home for emergencies.

Surviving Tornadoes and Hurricanes

Tornadoes are dangerous, funnel-shaped windstorms. They may strike and end quickly. Tornadoes can turn over cars. They can tear roofs off houses. They can tear large trees out of the ground.

During a tornado many people may be hurt or killed by flying objects. So it is best to stay in a basement or an inside hallway. If your house does not have a basement, stay on the first floor. Stay under a strong piece of furniture. Or stay in the bathtub, covered by a mattress or pillows. Stay away from windows. Go into a building for shelter if you are outdoors. Do not stay in a car or a mobile home.

Hurricanes are tropical storms with strong winds. They bring heavy rains that can cause floods. Sometimes they bring tornadoes. They can destroy buildings. They can damage electric and telephone lines.

You can prepare for a hurricane. Bring bikes, tools, lawn chairs, and garbage cans indoors. To prevent glass windows from breaking, nail wooden boards over them. You can also put wide strips of tape across them. Fill your tub and glass or plastic jars with fresh water. You can use this water if the storm damages the water supply. Sometimes people are told to **evacuate** their homes. They are told to wait in a safer place until the storm ends. Always follow these directions.

Surviving Lightning and Snowstorms

Lightning is electricity that is part of a thunderstorm. If lightning strikes you, you will get a strong electric shock. This shock can injure or kill you.

Stay indoors during a lightning storm. Unplug electric appliances when a storm starts. Try not to use the phone. Do not touch metal objects like stoves or sinks.

You can also protect yourself outdoors during a lightning storm. Tall objects **attract** lightning. So stay away from hills and trees. Find a low spot and lie down

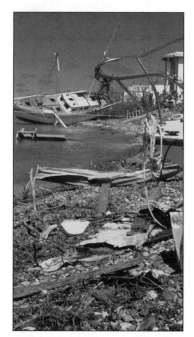

Hurricanes cause a lot of damage.

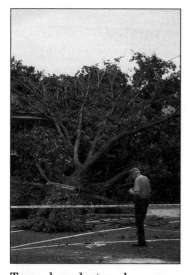

Tornadoes destroy houses and trees. Try to stay indoors in a basement during a tornado.

To **evacuate** means to leave.

To **attract** means to pull toward an object or person.

116

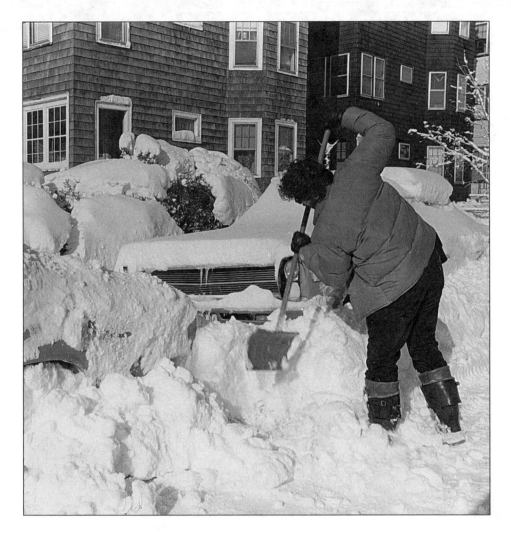

Try to stay at home during a blizzard. Cars may get stuck in snow.

on the ground. Electricity moves through water. So stay out of a swimming pool or the ocean. A car can be a safe place to wait during a lightning storm.

Blizzards are the most dangerous kind of snowstorm. Be safe during a blizzard. Stay inside your home. Have a supply of food and fresh, bottled water. Keep extra blankets in your car in case you are stuck there during a blizzard. If you are in a car, the storm may force you to stop. Wait on the right side of the road for help. Use the extra blankets to stay warm. Leave the light on inside your car. This will help others see the car, and you can be found.

You can help emergency workers. Stay away from emergency areas. Telephone lines must be kept open for emergency calls. So avoid using your phone. You can protect yourself during a natural disaster. Stay calm and remember what to do.

Using What You Learned

Vocabulary—Finish the Sentence

Choose a word or words from the box to complete each sentence. Write the correct answers on your paper.

evacuate	survive	natural disaster	attract

1. To _____ a disaster means to live through it.

2. Sometimes people must _____ their homes until a hurricane ends.

3. Tall objects _____ lightning.

4. A _____ is an accident caused by nature.

Comprehension—Write the Questions

Below are the answers for some questions from this chapter. Read each answer. Then write on your paper a possible question to go with each answer. Use the question words to help you.

1. Why _____ ?

   You will need batteries for a radio and a flashlight during emergencies.

2. Where _____ ?

   You should stay in a doorway between two rooms or sit under a strong desk or table during an earthquake.

3. What _____ ?

   Hurricanes are tropical storms with strong winds.

4. How _____ ?

   You can help emergency workers by staying away from emergency areas and by not using the telephone.

5. Where _____ ?

A safe place to wait during a lightning storm is inside a car.

6. What _____ ?

The most dangerous kind of snowstorm is a blizzard.

7. How _____ ?

Weather reports can be helpful because they warn about possible lightning storms, hurricanes, tornadoes, and snowstorms.

Critical Thinking—Cause and Effect

Write sentences on your paper by matching each cause on the left with an effect on the right.

Cause

1. A natural disaster has hit your area, so _____

2. An earthquake shakes and cracks the ground, so _____

3. You are caught outside during a lightning storm, so _____

4. You want to be prepared for a natural disaster, so _____

5. You are in your car during a blizzard, so _____

6. Your house does not have a basement, so _____

Effect

a. you find a low spot and lie down on the ground.

b. you do not have electricity or running water in your house.

c. you store a radio, a flashlight, canned food, and other emergency supplies.

d. buildings, bridges, and highways fall down.

e. during a tornado you stay in an inside hallway.

f. you stop on the right side of the road and use blankets to stay warm.

UNIT 6

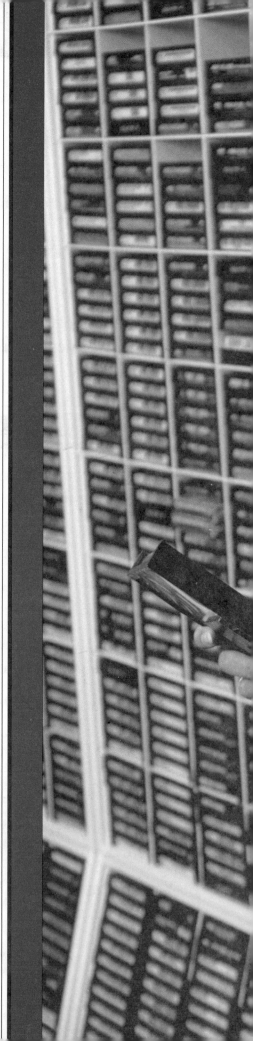

Consumer Health

You make many decisions when you shop. You decide what to buy and how much money to spend. You decide if what you buy is safe. You also make decisions when you need health care. You decide when you need checkups and which doctor to visit.

You must learn how to make wise decisions when you shop. By studying about health care goods and services, you can learn to make health decisions wisely.

Have You Ever Wondered?

▼ You can learn to spend your money wisely. How?
▼ Many people do not visit skilled doctors for their health problems. Why?
▼ All people need regular checkups. Why?

As you read this unit, think about how you can spend your money wisely. Learning how to make wise choices will help you reach your goal of wellness.

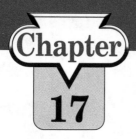
Becoming a Wise Consumer

Think About as You Read

- How can peer pressure affect consumers?
- How can knowing the unit price help consumers?
- How do ads affect consumers?

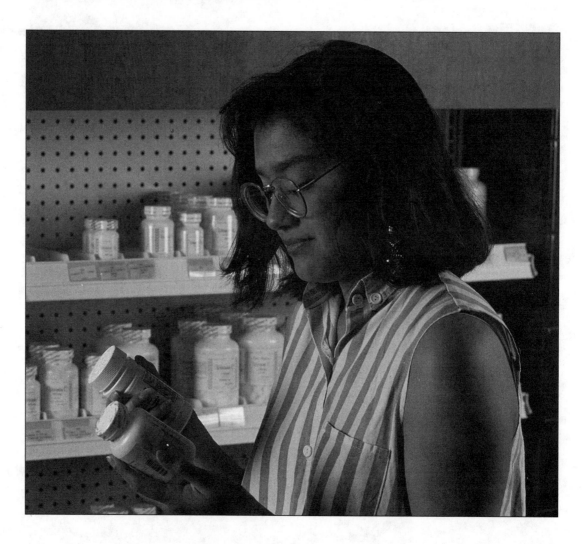

Make wise
decisions when
you shop.

Jason needed shampoo for his hair. He found ten
kinds of shampoo in the store. Jason knew that all
shampoos can clean hair. He bought the cheapest one.
He was not sure whether he made the right choice.

122

Being a Wise Consumer

Every person who buys and uses a **product** or service is a **consumer**. A consumer's goal is to spend money wisely.

A **budget** can help you manage your money. Know how much money you have. Then decide how to spend it wisely.

Think about what you need to buy. Make a shopping list before you go to the store. Buy the things that are on your list when you shop.

How can you decide which products or services to buy? Sometimes you can find out about products and services from **ads**. You can ask your family and friends about the products and services they use. You can also learn about products and services by reading consumer magazines. They tell about many kinds of products and services.

A **product** is anything that is made.

A **budget** is a plan for spending money.

Ads tell what is special or good about a product or service.

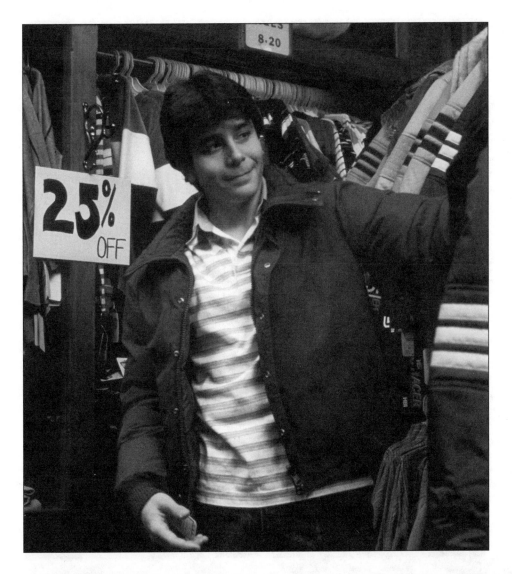

Know how much money is in your budget. Then you can decide how much to spend.

You can be a wise consumer and save money. Compare the prices of products in a few stores. Then buy the product in the store where it is cheapest.

Peer pressure can stop you from being a wise consumer. To feel accepted by your friends, you may think you need to wear the same kind of clothes, shoes, and make-up they wear. You may spend too much money on products that are not right for you.

Teens often feel pressure to buy **fad** clothing. These clothes are in style for only a short time. Many people will not wear clothes that are no longer in style. Avoid buying fad clothing.

What Is a Unit Price?

The **unit price** is the price of one ounce, pound, quart, or other measurement of a product.

You can use the **unit price** to compare prices on similar products. To learn the unit price, divide the price by the weight of the product. For example, a

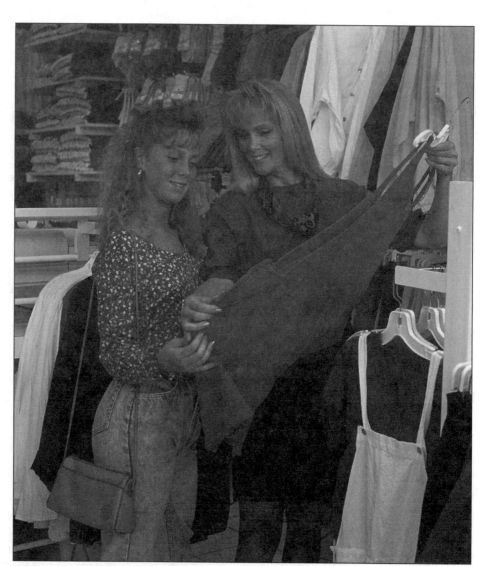

Compare prices in a few stores. Then buy products you like with the best prices.

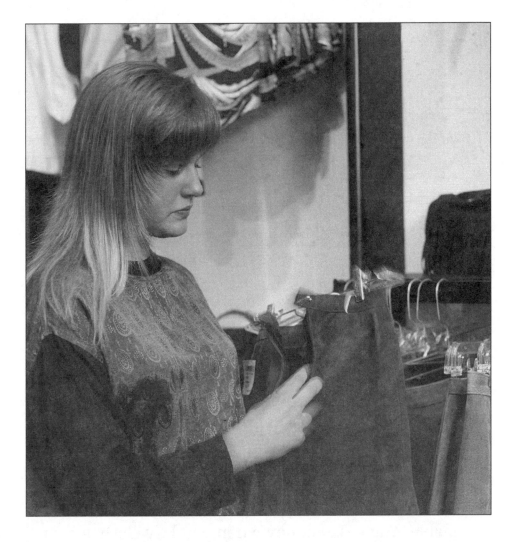

You should always read the labels on clothes before you buy them.

five-ounce tube of toothpaste costs two dollars. Its unit price is 40 cents.

Often the unit price is lower for the larger sizes of a product. You may save money if you buy the largest size. But you may not need the largest size. Then buy a smaller size even if its unit price is higher.

How to Buy Products Wisely

We all use health care products. Some health care products are soaps, sunscreens, and shampoos. You use health care products to improve your health, treat an illness, or stay well. When you try a new health care product, always buy the smallest size. If you like the health care product, buy a larger size when you need it.

Always read the labels on clothes before you buy them. The label tells you directions for how to care for the clothes. Some clothes must be dry-cleaned. This is

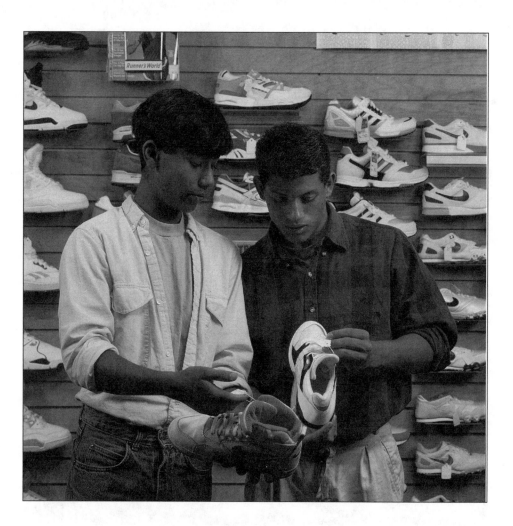

Buy shoes that fit well and feel comfortable. Expensive shoes are not always the best.

expensive. You save money when you buy clothes that you can wash.

Always buy shoes that fit well. Have both feet measured when you buy shoes. Expensive shoes are not always better than cheaper ones.

Ask yourself these questions when you shop.
1. Why am I buying this? Do I really need it?
2. What is the best choice?
3. Do I have enough money to buy this?

Tina found two pairs of jeans that fit well. One pair was very expensive, but all of her friends had a pair just like it. The other pair was cheaper, but it was made well. Tina decided to buy the cheaper pair. She knew this was a wise way to spend her money.

Understanding Ads

The companies that make products want you to buy their products. You see ads in newspapers and magazines. You see them on TV and hear them on the radio. Ads provide the consumer with facts about a product or a service.

Some ads try to make you feel that you need a product so that you will buy it. Ads may do this in five different ways.

1. A free gift is given away with each product that is bought.
2. Ads will say that everyone is using this product.
3. Ads will say that doctors and hospitals use this product.
4. Ads will use a famous person to tell about a product or service. This kind of ad should make you want to use the product or service, too.
5. Ads will say that you deserve the best, most expensive product.

Buy products that you really need. Choose carefully. Do not spend more money than your budget allows. Then you will be a better consumer.

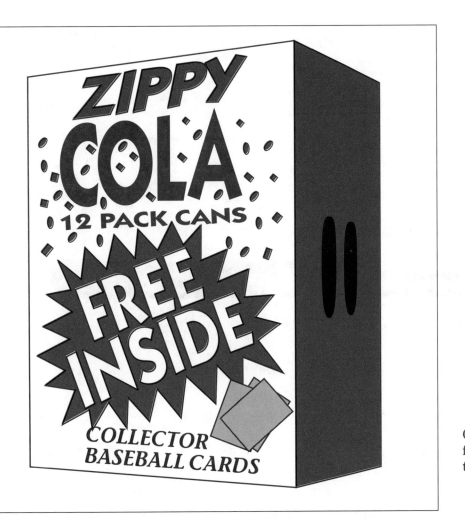

Companies may give away free gifts to people who buy their products.

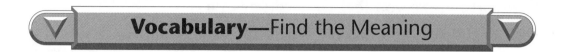
Using What You Learned

Write on your paper the word or words that best complete each sentence.

1. A plan you make for how you will spend your money is a _____ .

   fad   **product**   **budget**

2. You are a _____ when you buy and use a product or service.

   budget   **consumer**   **peer**

3. You divide the amount that a product costs by its weight to find its
   _____ .

   free gift   **ad**   **unit price**

4. A company may use _____ to make you want to use its product or
   service.

   ads   **peers**   **budgets**

5. The thing that you buy is a _____ .

   goal   **product**   **consumer**

6. You should avoid buying _____ clothing because it is in style for only a
   short time.

   fad   **ads**   **dry-clean**

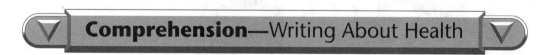
Comprehension—Writing About Health

Answer the following question in complete sentences on your paper.

What are three things you can do to be a wise consumer?

Critical Thinking—Fact or Opinion

Write **Fact** on your paper for each fact below. Write **Opinion** for each opinion. You should find five sentences that are opinions.

1. Many consumers try to spend their money wisely.

2. It is easier to buy a product than it is to choose a service.

3. A budget shows how much money you have and how you plan to spend that money.

4. Reading consumer magazines is the best way to find out about a product.

5. Peer pressure can make you spend too much money on products that are not right for you.

6. Toothpaste, soap, and deodorant are types of health care products.

7. Labels tell you how to take care of your clothes.

8. Fad clothes are only in style for a little while.

9. Expensive clothes are always made better than cheaper ones.

10. Some ads use a famous person to tell you about a product.

11. It is easy to ignore peer pressure when you are deciding what products to buy.

12. You can save money by comparing prices at different stores.

13. Ads are used to provide the consumer with facts about a product or service.

14. It is always a good idea to buy the largest size of a product.

Chapter 18

Protecting the Consumer

Think About as You Read

- **Why should you avoid quackery?**
- **How does the government protect consumers?**
- **How can consumers protect themselves?**

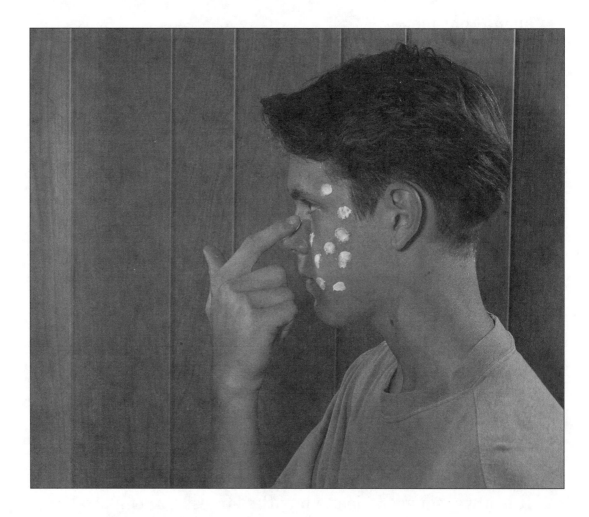

Many people spend money on useless products that are supposed to work miracles.

Miracles are things that cannot be explained.

Quackery is the selling of useless health products and services.

Chang had acne. One day he saw an ad for an acne medicine. It was supposed to work **miracles**. Chang ordered the new medicine. He used it every day. But his acne only got worse. Chang knew he had wasted his money on **quackery**.

As you read this chapter, you will learn how quackery hurts consumers. You will also learn how consumers are protected from quackery.

Understanding Quackery

Quackery is the selling of health care products that do not work. These products, such as pills, things to wear, or special diets, are useless. A **quack** is a person who tries to sell you useless health care products and services.

Why do many people go to quacks instead of skilled doctors? Some people are fooled by quackery. They want to look better quickly. They want clear, smooth skin. They want to lose weight quickly. They want to look younger and thinner.

Other people visit quacks to be treated for real health problems. A disease like **arthritis** can be

Arthritis is a disease that causes pain and stiffness in the body's joints.

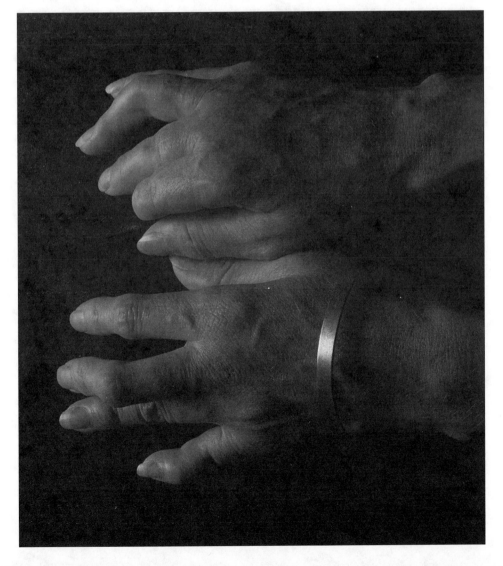

Many people believe wearing a copper bracelet will cure arthritis.

controlled with medicine. But it cannot be cured. Yet some people hope these quacks will cure the disease.

Other people use quacks because they do not want to spend the time or money going to doctors. They do not want to take real medical tests. Many people use quacks because they do not want to learn new, healthier habits.

Avoiding Quackery

Avoid quackery because it can be dangerous. Quackery often uses products and services that are not safe. Sometimes people go to quacks, and they do not get the medical treatment they need. Without treatment, diseases such as cancer get worse quickly.

Every year Americans spend millions of dollars on quackery. When these people need real medical care, they do not have the money for it.

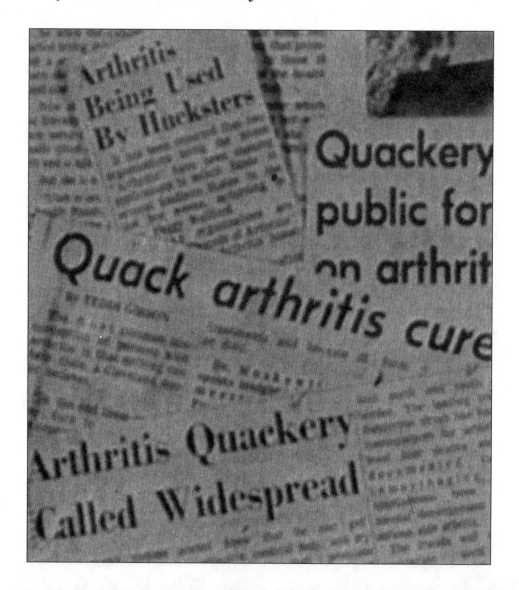

People spend millions of dollars on quackery.

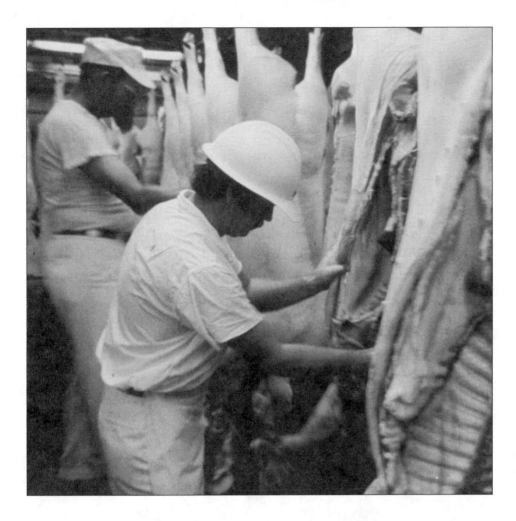

The FDA checks companies to make sure food products are safe for consumers.

You can avoid quackery. First, pay attention to the words used in ads. Quackery ads promise quick, easy cures or changes. Second, read newspapers or magazines to learn about new products. Third, remember that most health problems do not have fast, easy answers. Fourth, discuss health care products that you have questions about with your doctor or school nurse.

The Government Protects Consumers

Three **agencies** protect you as a consumer.
1. The Food and Drug Administration (FDA) checks to make sure that companies sell safe food, health care products, medicines, and **cosmetics**.
2. The Federal Trade Commission (FTC) protects against false advertising. It tries to make sure that ads do not make untrue statements about a product or service.

Agencies are government offices that do certain kinds of work.

Cosmetics are products that are used to make the face, hair, or some other part of the body look more beautiful.

3. The Consumer Product Safety Commission (CPSC) gives consumers facts about the safety of products.

More Protection for Consumers

Two other groups of people also help consumers. One group is Underwriters Laboratories. It tests the safety of many electrical products. Products that pass these safety tests have a UL label.

The Consumer Union helps consumers. It tests and compares products. This group prepares a consumer magazine.

As a consumer you can protect yourself. Pay close attention to warnings on product labels. Always read and follow the directions on these labels. Read ads carefully. Avoid health quackery.

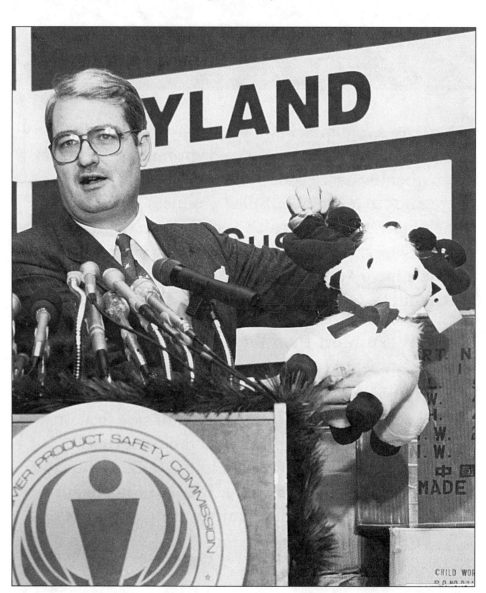

The Consumer Product Safety Commission can give you facts about the safety of products.

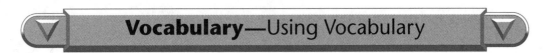

Vocabulary—Using Vocabulary

Use the word or words to write a complete sentence on your paper about quackery.

1. miracles
2. quack
3. agencies
4. arthritis
5. medical treatment

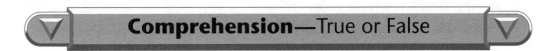

Comprehension—True or False

Write **True** on your paper for each sentence that is true. Write **False** on your paper for each sentence that is false. There are four false sentences. Rewrite the false sentences on your paper to make them true.

1. Quackery is the selling of health care products that work.

2. A person who tries to sell you useless health care products and services is called a quack.

3. You should discuss health care products that you have questions about with your doctor or school nurse.

4. The Food and Drug Administration protects consumers against false advertising.

5. The Consumer Union tests and compares products.

6. People with diseases like arthritis cannot be fooled by quackery.

7. People usually go to quacks because they want to look better slowly.

8. Every year Americans spend millions of dollars on quackery.

9. Ads that promise quick, easy cures or changes usually are quackery ads.

10. Consumers can protect themselves by carefully reading warnings on product labels.

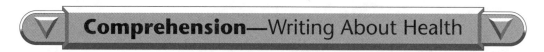

Comprehension—Writing About Health

Answer the following question in complete sentences on your paper.

Why do many people go to quacks instead of to skilled doctors?

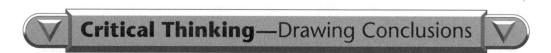

Critical Thinking—Drawing Conclusions

Read the paragraph. Then use the six steps to decide what to do about buying a new shampoo for oily hair. Write complete sentences on your paper to answer each question.

> You have very oily hair. You wash your hair every day, but it doesn't seem to help. You have seen some ads for a new shampoo that cures the problem of oily hair after one use. But this new shampoo is very expensive.

Step 1. What is the problem?

Step 2. What are two ways to solve the problem?

Step 3. What is one consequence for each choice listed in Step 2?

Step 4. Which choice do you think is best?

Step 5. What can you do to put your decision into action?

Step 6. Think about your decision. Why was this the best choice for you?

Choosing Health Care

Think About as You Read

- What should your personal health records show?
- Why are health checkups important?
- How can people pay for health care?

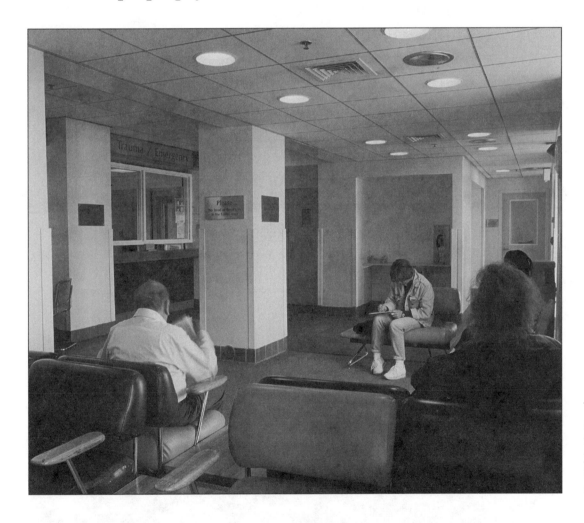

You can get emergency treatment from your doctor or from a hospital emergency room.

Matthew broke his finger. Matthew knew he could go to his doctor. He could also go to the hospital emergency room to get help. Every person must know how to get good health care. Good health care helps us reach the goal of wellness.

Being a Wise Health Care Consumer

Choose your doctor and dentist before you have health problems. You can find a doctor or dentist by asking someone you know to suggest one. You can also ask another doctor or nurse to suggest one.

Many people get health care from health **clinics**. They use clinics because they pay only what they can afford.

You should keep personal health records. Your records should show seven things.

1. Changes in your height and weight
2. Dates of **immunization** shots
3. Dates of other checkups
4. Dates of illnesses
5. Dates of **surgery** and other hospital stays
6. **Allergies** to food and medicine
7. Family health problems

Your Medical Checkup

Do not wait until you are sick to see a doctor. Have a checkup every year. A checkup helps you find and take care of small health problems before they become big ones. Add your checkup to your personal health records.

Clinics are places where doctors and nurses treat health problems.

An **immunization** is a type of medicine that stops a person from getting a disease.

Surgery is the use of medical tools to operate on the body.

Allergies cause a person to have a runny or stuffy nose, have breathing problems, or have other health problems. Allergies are caused by certain foods, plants, or other things that don't bother many other people.

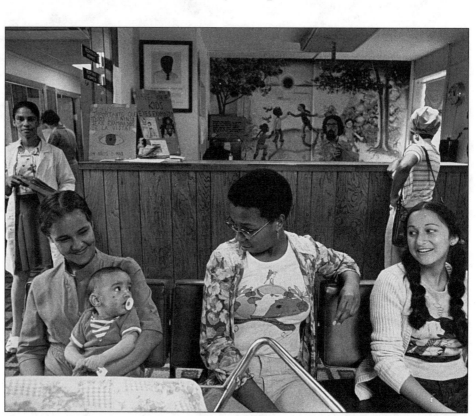

Many people go to clinics for health care. People pay only what they can afford.

138

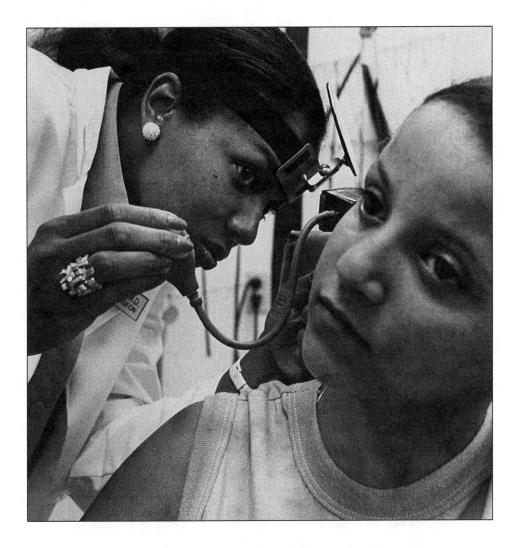

Everyone needs checkups. Talk to your doctor about your health questions.

During a checkup the doctor will ask about your health history. Tell the doctor about any changes in your personal health records. Talk to your doctor about any health questions that are worrying you.

Buying Medicine Wisely

Buy your medicine at a drugstore where you can talk to a **pharmacist**. Ask questions about your medicine. Should you take it after meals? Will this medicine make you sleepy?

Follow your doctor's directions when taking all medicine. Take your medicine for the number of days that your doctor has ordered.

People often save money when they buy a **generic** medicine. When you need to take a medicine, ask your doctor or pharmacist if you can buy the generic medicine.

A **pharmacist** is a person who prepares medicine your doctor has ordered for you.

Generic means a product has the same purpose and ingredients as a product with a company name. A generic product usually costs less.

139

Paying for Health Care

Health care is expensive. Most people need health insurance to help them pay for their health care.

The government has two health insurance programs. **Medicare** pays for hospital stays of people who are at least 65 years old. Young people with **disabilities** can also receive Medicare. **Medicaid** helps people who do not earn much money. Medicaid pays for visits to clinics. It pays for hospital stays. It also pays for medicines and certain doctor bills.

Many people pay for their own health insurance. There are three kinds of health insurance people pay for. **Hospitalization** pays for part of the cost of staying in a hospital. Medical insurance helps pay for doctors' services, medicines, and some health tests. **Major medical** helps pay for very large health bills. It pays for surgery and expensive health tests.

Many people pay for health care by joining a **health maintenance organization**, or HMO. People pay to be members of the HMO. The HMO then offers most health services at a special rate. Members must use the HMO's doctors, hospitals, and clinics.

Make good decisions for your own health care. Choose your doctors and dentists wisely. Take care of your health to feel your best each day.

Disabilities limit people's ability to do such things as walk, lift, hear, see, or learn.

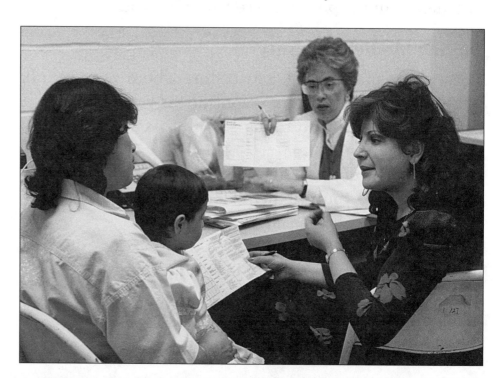

There are many kinds of health insurance. Insurance helps people pay for health care.

Using What You Learned

Vocabulary—Matching

Match each vocabulary word in **Group B** with a sentence from **Group A** that tells about the word. Write the letter of the correct answer on your paper.

Group A

1. This product has the same purpose and ingredients as a product with a company name, but it usually costs less.

2. This is the use of medical tools to operate on the body.

3. Doctors provide health care here, and patients pay only what they can afford.

4. This government insurance pays some of the health care expenses for people who do not earn much money.

5. This insurance pays part of the cost of being in the hospital.

Group B

a. Medicaid

b. surgery

c. hospitalization

d. clinic

e. generic

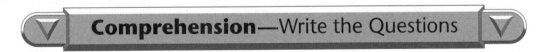

Comprehension—Write the Questions

Below are the answers for some questions from this chapter. Read each answer. Then write on your paper a possible question to go with each answer. Use the question words to help you.

1. When _____ ?

   You should choose your doctor or dentist before you have health problems.

2. Where _____ ?

   You can go to health clinics to get health care at a price you can afford.

3. How _____ ?

You should go to your doctor for a checkup every year.

4. Who _____ ?

Your doctor can answer any health questions that are worrying you.

5. Who _____ ?

Your doctor or pharmacist knows about generic medicines.

6. How _____ ?

The government has two health insurance programs.

7. What _____ ?

Major medical is insurance that helps pay for very large health bills.

Critical Thinking—Analogies

Use a word in the box to finish each sentence. Write the correct answers on your paper.

immunizations	Medicaid	pharmacists	surgery	dentist	HMO

1. Medical insurance is to doctors' services as major medical is to _____ .

2. Health care is to doctors as medicine is to _____ .

3. Government is to Medicaid as member is to _____ .

4. Physical health is to a doctor as dental health is to a _____ .

5. Medical tools for operating are to surgery as shots are to _____ .

6. Age is to Medicare as money earned is to _____ .

Read the words in each group. Decide how they are alike. Find the best title in the box for each group. Write the title on your paper.

Wise Consumer	**Allergies**	**Personal Health Records**
Health Checkup	**Pharmacist**	**Health Insurance**

1. dates of immunization shots
   allergies to foods and medicines
   changes in height and weight

2. prevents serious health problems
   needed every year
   a time to ask health questions

3. works at a drugstore
   answers questions about medicine
   prepares medicines ordered by a doctor

4. may cause breathing problems
   may be caused by foods or plants
   do not bother everyone

5. chooses a doctor while healthy
   asks questions about medicines
   plans how to pay for health care

6. Medicare and Medicaid
   helps pay for surgery
   helps pay for medicines

UNIT 7

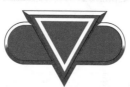

Growth and Development

Imagine being a member of a band. To be a great band, all the players and their instruments must work together. Like the band the parts of your body must work together so you can be healthy.

The parts of your body depend on each other. Strong bones and muscles allow you to move easily. Exercise makes your heart stronger. A strong, healthy heart can pump blood easily to every part of the body.

Have You Ever Wondered?

▼ Your bones cannot move without your muscles. How do muscles move bones?
▼ Your body has red blood cells and white blood cells. Why does it need both?
▼ You can breathe with your nose and with your mouth. It is healthier to breathe with your nose. Why?

As you read this unit, think of ways you can keep the parts of your body healthy so they can work together for you.

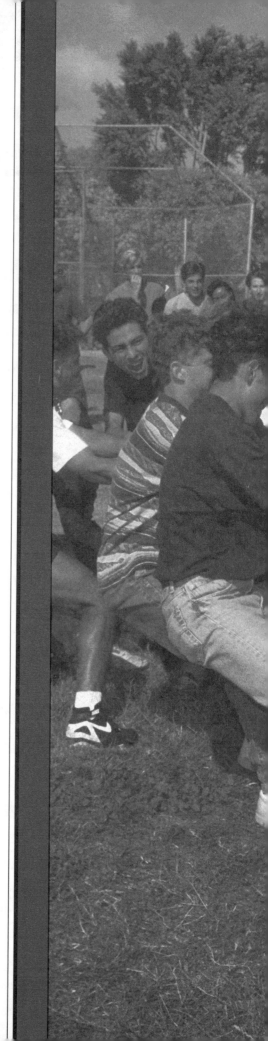

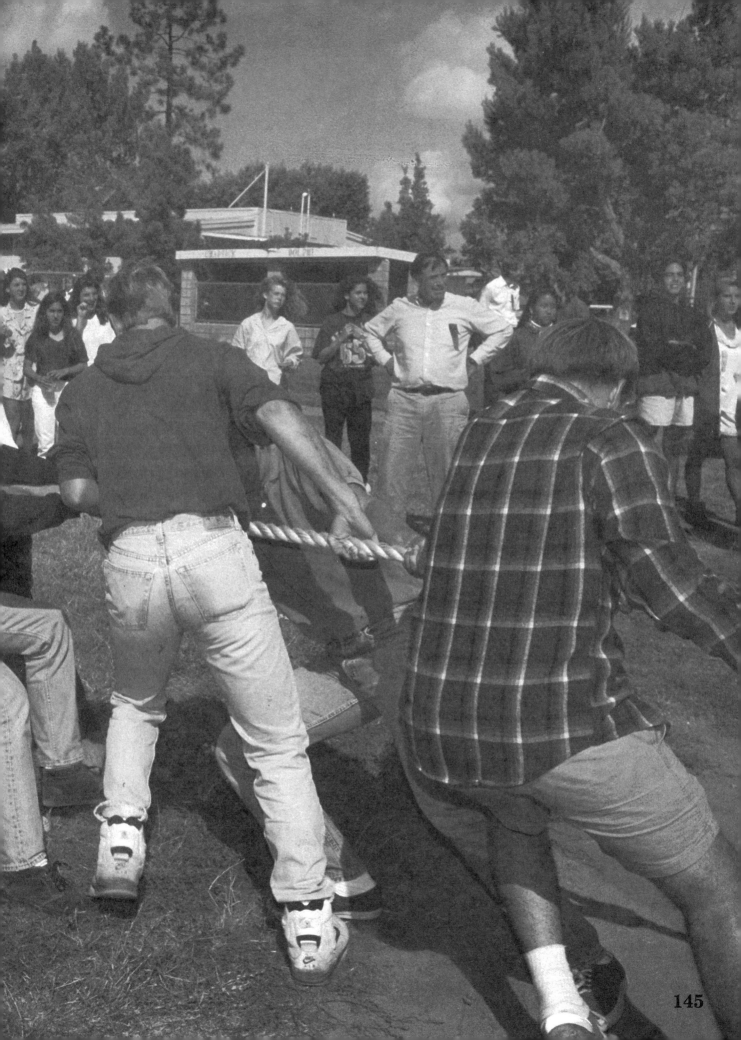

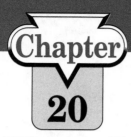

Chapter
20

Your Cells, Bones, and Muscles

Think About as You Read

- How do bones and muscles help you move?
- How can you have good posture?
- How can you build strong bones and muscles?

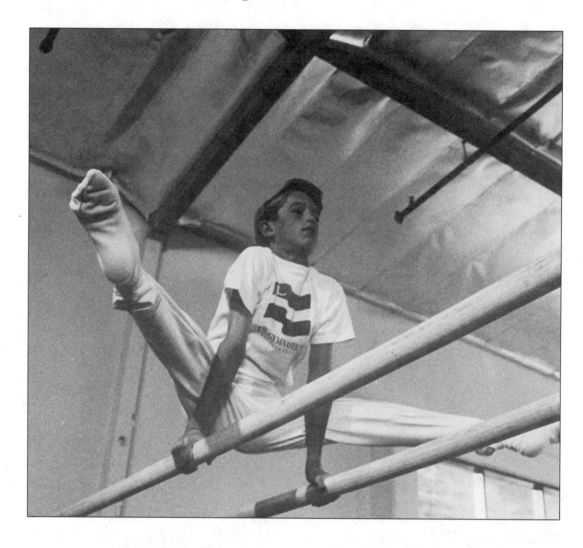

Your body can move in many ways. It moves because you have bones and muscles.

Your body is always moving. It moves when you run and jump. It also moves when you turn over while you sleep. Your body can move because you have bones and muscles.

Millions of Cells

Cells are very tiny living things. All plants and animals are made of cells. You cannot see the cells of your body because the cells are too small. Every cell of the body must have food and **oxygen**.

The body has many kinds of cells. Some of the different cells are the blood cells, skin cells, and muscle cells. Large groups of cells form **organs** inside your body. Your heart, brain, and stomach are three organs. Groups of organs work together to form the body's **systems**.

Oxygen is a gas that has no color or smell.

Your Bones

Your body has more than 200 bones. The bones help you in four ways. First, your bones keep all of the other parts of your body in place so you can stand and sit. Second, your bones work with your muscles to help you move. Third, blood cells are made inside your bones. Fourth, your bones protect the organs inside your body. For example, your ribs protect your heart.

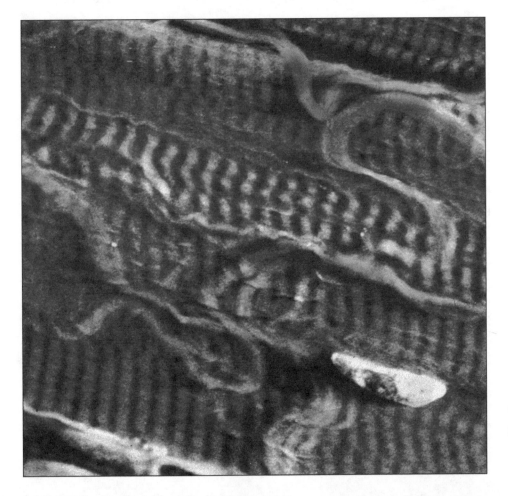

These are muscle cells as seen through a microscope.

147

Your body has three kinds of bones. You have long bones in your arms and legs. You have short bones in your hands, fingers, and spine. Flat bones protect your brain. The ribs around your heart are also flat bones.

Your bones fit together at **joints**. Some joints help you move. Your arms, legs, toes, and neck have joints so they can move. The bones that protect your brain and your heart have joints that do not move.

Your Muscles

Your body has more than 600 muscles. You have muscles all over your body. Skin covers your muscles. Small muscles allow you to move your eyes, lips, and tongue. Large muscles allow you to move your arms and legs.

Your body has two types of muscles. **Voluntary muscles** allow you to move. You can control your voluntary muscles. They are attached to the arms, legs, and spine. They are also attached to the other bones that move. Voluntary muscles work in pairs. To move a bone, one muscle pulls the bone while the other muscle relaxes.

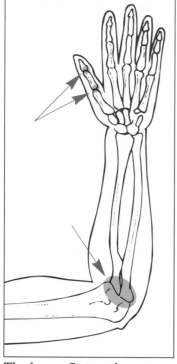

The bones fit together at joints. The arrows show a joint at the elbow and two joints in the thumb.

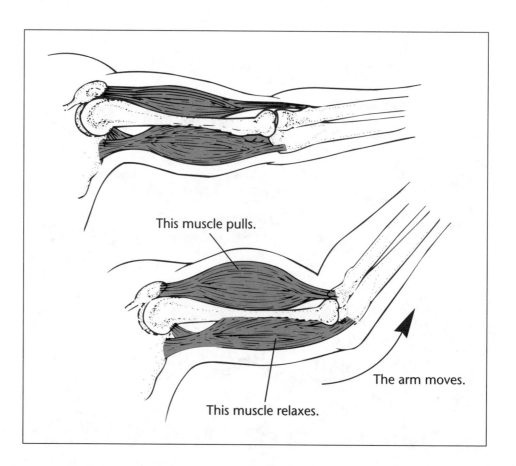

This muscle pulls.

The arm moves.

This muscle relaxes.

Muscles relax and pull to make your arm move.

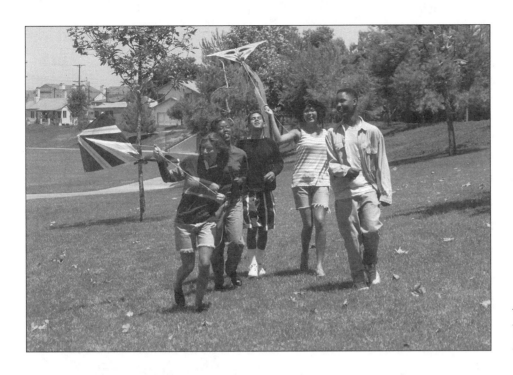

You can stand and move because you have bones and muscles.

Involuntary muscles control your heart and your breathing. They keep your stomach working. Your brain sends messages to these muscles. With these messages the muscles can work on their own. These muscles keep working even while you sleep.

Taking Care of Your Bones and Muscles

Your posture is the way you carry your body when you sit, stand, and walk. You must use your bones and muscles to stand and sit correctly.

Why do you need good posture? Good posture helps your appearance. It also helps your bones and muscles grow the way they should. Also, good posture keeps your organs in their correct places inside your body.

There are three causes of poor posture. The first is poor standing and sitting habits. Many people do not work at having good standing and sitting habits. The lack of strong muscles in your back and stomach area is the second cause. The third cause is a health problem called **scoliosis**. Scoliosis is an unhealthy curving of the spine. Your school nurse or doctor can check your back for scoliosis during a checkup. It should be treated when it is found in teen-agers. Scoliosis can cause other health problems.

You can have good posture. Practice standing and sitting correctly. Do exercises to make the muscles in your back and around your stomach stronger.

To build strong bones and muscles, exercise at least three times a week. Walk, run, jog, or play tennis. Jumping rope and lifting weights also make your bones and muscles stronger. Stretching exercises help arms and legs bend and move easily. As you grow older, you should continue to do stretching exercises as well as exercises to build your bones and muscles.

Lifting objects correctly is a way to care for your back. Always lift objects by bending at your knees. Keep your back straight.

Osteoporosis is a bone disease that can affect older adults. To protect yourself from this disease, eat enough foods with calcium. Milk, cheese, and dark green vegetables have lots of calcium. Do exercises that build strong bones.

You use your bones and muscles to move. You must take care of them by having good posture habits. Eat foods with calcium every day and exercise at least three times a week. Caring for your bones and muscles will help you have a healthy body.

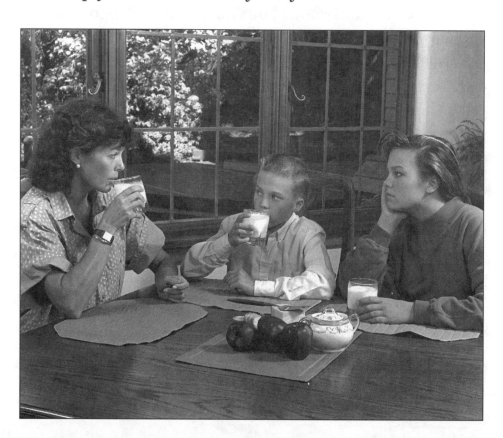

Milk, cheese, and dark green vegetables are rich in calcium. Eat them to have healthy bones.

Using What You Learned

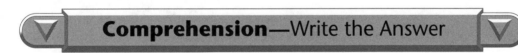
Vocabulary—Matching

Match each vocabulary word in **Group B** with a sentence from **Group A** that tells about the word. Write the letter of the correct answer on your paper.

Group A

1. These are formed by large groups of cells.

2. This is a gas that is needed by every cell of the body.

3. These are places in the body where bones fit together.

4. These are formed by groups of organs that work together.

5. These muscles control your heart and your breathing.

6. These muscles allow you to move.

Group B

a. oxygen

b. systems

c. involuntary muscles

d. organs

e. joints

f. voluntary muscles

Comprehension—Write the Answer

Write a sentence on your paper to answer each question.

1. Why can't you see the cells in your body?

2. Which bones protect your heart?

3. What is scoliosis?

4. How often should you exercise to build strong bones and muscles?

5. How do voluntary muscles work?

6. What must every cell of the body have?

Critical Thinking—Fact or Opinion

Write **Fact** on your paper for each fact below. Write **Opinion** for each opinion. You should find two sentences that are opinions.

1. The human body has three kinds of bones.

2. Involuntary muscles control your breathing.

3. Foods that are rich in calcium taste good.

4. Good posture helps bones and muscles grow the way they should.

5. Running is the best form of exercise.

6. Eating foods with calcium can help prevent osteoporosis.

Critical Thinking—Categories

Read the words in each group. Decide how they are alike. Find the best title in the box for each group. Write the title on your paper.

Involuntary Muscles	Good Posture
Cells	Bones

1. found in all living things
   too small to see
   need food and oxygen

2. can be long, short, or flat
   help you move
   protect your organs

3. control your heart and breathing
   keep your stomach working
   work even while you are sleeping

4. helps your appearance
   keeps your organs in the correct
      places
   helps your bones and muscles grow
      correctly

152

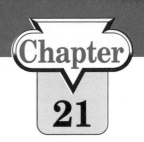

The Digestive and Circulatory Systems

Think About as You Read

- What happens to food in the digestive system?
- How does blood move through your body?
- How can you care for your digestive and circulatory systems?

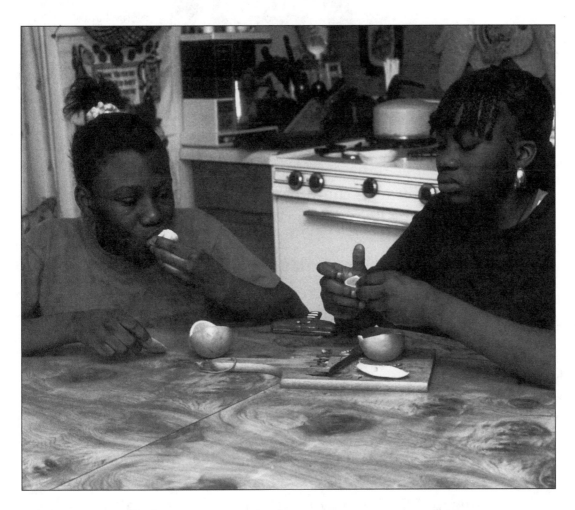

Fruits and vegetables are healthy foods. They have many nutrients that your body needs.

Every cell in your body must have oxygen. Every cell also needs nutrients from the food you eat. Your body breaks down food so your cells can get nutrients. Your blood carries the nutrients and oxygen to every cell of the body.

153

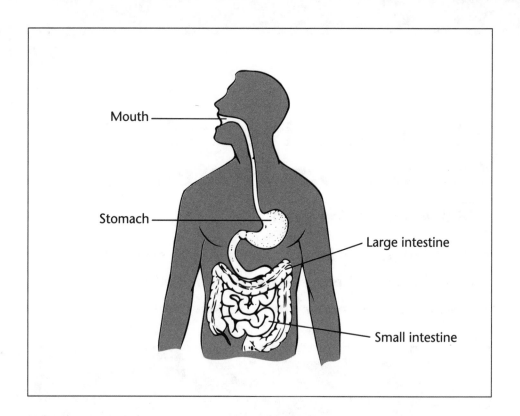

The organs of the digestive system break down food so it can be used by your cells.

Digestion is the way the body breaks down your food into nutrients the body can use.

Enzymes are chemicals made by the body and used to break down food.

The Work of the Digestive System

The food that you eat must be changed so its nutrients can be used by the body. Your body has a group of organs that breaks down food so it can be used by the body. These organs form your **digestive system**.

Digestion begins in the mouth. Your teeth chew food into small pieces. As you chew, **enzymes** in your mouth begin to break down the food.

Food passes from the mouth through a long tube and enters your stomach. Muscles and enzymes in the stomach break down the food further. After food is digested by the stomach, it then passes into the **small intestine**.

The small intestine finishes most of the job of digestion. More enzymes break down the food. The digested food is now ready to leave the small intestine. This digested food looks like thin soup. Now the body's cells can use the digested food.

Digested food passes through the walls of the small intestine into the blood. Then your blood carries nutrients from the digested food to every cell.

Digestion cannot break down some foods, like fruit skins. Foods that cannot be digested become solid waste. The **large intestine** stores solid waste until the solid waste leaves the body.

The Circulatory System

The **circulatory system** has three parts. The three parts are the heart, the blood, and the **blood vessels**. Arteries, **veins**, and **capillaries** are the three types of blood vessels in the body.

The job of the circulatory system is to bring food and oxygen to every part of the body. To do this job, the heart pumps blood. Then blood vessels carry blood to every cell of the body. Then other blood vessels carry blood back to the heart. This happens thousands of times each day. The heart never stops pumping while a person is alive.

Blood vessels are the different kinds of tubes that carry blood throughout the body.

Veins are blood vessels that carry blood from other parts of the body back to the heart.

Capillaries are very tiny blood vessels that connect arteries and veins. Capillaries carry blood, oxygen, and nutrients to the body cells.

The Circulatory System

vein

lungs

artery

heart

Your heart pumps all the time. Blood vessels carry blood to every cell in your body.

How Blood Moves Through the Body

Your circulatory system moves your blood throughout your body.

1. The right side of the heart pumps blood with **carbon dioxide** to the lungs.
2. Blood gets oxygen and loses carbon dioxide at the lungs.
3. Blood leaves the lungs and is pumped to the left side of the heart.
4. The left side of the heart pumps blood into the arteries. The arteries divide into smaller blood vessels called capillaries. The capillaries carry blood to the body cells.
5. Capillaries bring oxygen and nutrients to the body cells. Capillaries pick up carbon dioxide and waste.
6. Capillaries join to form larger blood vessels called veins. Veins carry carbon dioxide to the right side of the heart.

When cells use nutrients and oxygen, they make a gas called **carbon dioxide**. Carbon dioxide leaves the body when you breathe out.

Arteries, capillaries, and veins are the three kinds of blood vessels.

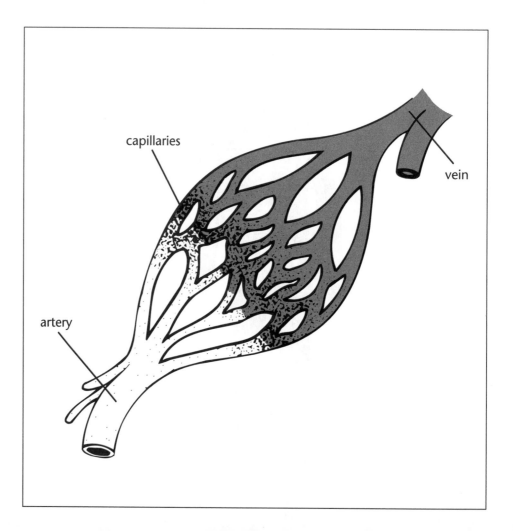

156

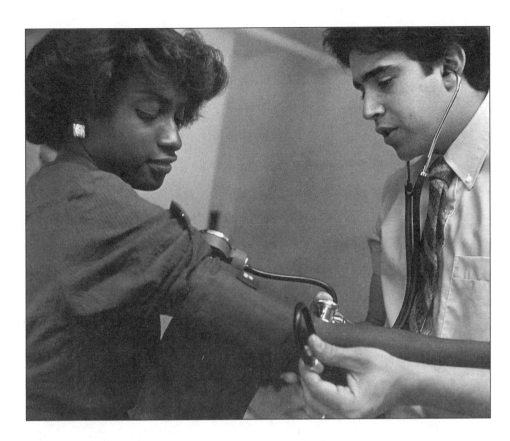

Your doctor should check your blood pressure when you have a checkup.

Your Blood and Your Blood Pressure

Your blood has red blood cells and white blood cells. Both kinds of blood cells are made inside your bones. You have more red blood cells than white blood cells. The red blood cells carry oxygen. The white blood cells help your body fight germs. You would be sick most of the time if you did not have white blood cells.

Your blood pressure is the force of your blood as it moves against the walls of the arteries or the heart. The arteries can stretch to become larger or smaller. This helps the blood flow through the arteries.

Some people have a health problem called high blood pressure. High blood pressure occurs for many reasons. People with high blood pressure have overworked hearts. High blood pressure can cause tiny blood vessels to burst. This can damage body organs, such as the brain. High blood pressure can also lead to heart disease or other body organ diseases. Your doctor should check your blood pressure when you have a checkup. A healthy diet, exercise, and medicine can help treat high blood pressure.

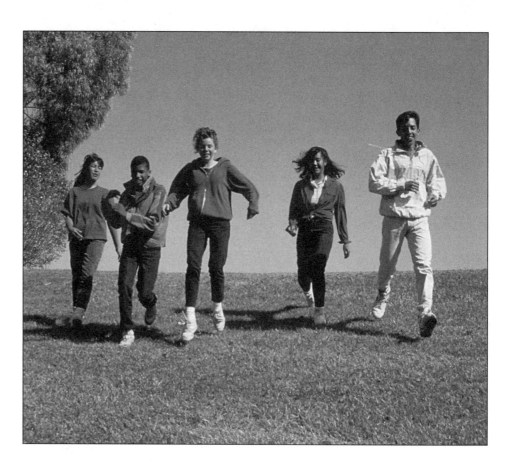

To have a healthy heart, exercise at least three times a week. Eat less fat and salt.

Caring for Your Digestive and Circulatory Systems

Follow these five rules to keep your systems healthy.

1. Exercise at least three times a week. Exercise makes your heart and arteries stronger. It helps lower your blood pressure.
2. Do not smoke or use drugs in ways that are not correct. Do not drink alcohol.
3. Control your weight. Do not eat more food than you need. Your heart must work much harder if you are overweight.
4. Eat a healthy diet. Eat many fruits and vegetables. Your diet should be low in fat and salt. Eat less fried food, egg yolks, and red meat. Drink skim milk instead of whole milk.
5. See your doctor for regular checkups. If you have high blood pressure, it should be treated.

Take care of your body's systems. Caring for your body's systems will help you have a healthy body.

158

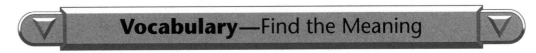

Using What You Learned

Vocabulary—Find the Meaning

Write on your paper the word or words that best complete each sentence.

1. The _____ system is the group of organs that break down food so it can be used by the body.

   circulatory   **digestive**   **bone**

2. The gas made by cells when they use nutrients and oxygen is _____ .

   small intestine   **blood**   **carbon dioxide**

3. The _____ carry blood to the heart.

   veins   **enzymes**   **nutrients**

4. The _____ stores solid waste.

   capillary   **large intestine**   **heart**

5. The chemicals in the body that help break down food are _____ .

   enzymes   **wastes**   **oxygen**

6. The _____ system brings food and oxygen to every part of the body.

   circulatory   **digestive**   **bone**

7. Food that is digested by the stomach is passed into the _____ .

   small intestine   **enzymes**   **nutrients**

8. The _____ connect arteries and veins.

   enzymes   **white blood cells** **capillaries**

9. The three parts of the circulatory system are the heart, blood, and _____ .

   lungs   **blood vessels**   **intestines**

159

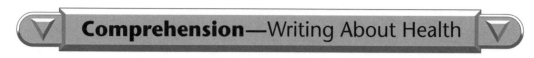

Comprehension—Writing About Health

Answer the following question in complete sentences on your paper.

What are three things you can do to care for your digestive and circulatory systems?

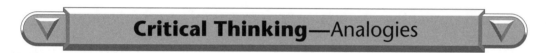

Critical Thinking—Analogies

Use a word or words in the box to finish each sentence. Write the correct answers on your paper.

nutrients	veins	circulatory system	large intestine
solid wastes	mouth	white blood cells	exercise

1. The small intestine is to finishing digestion as the _____ is to beginning digestion.

2. The digestive system is to food as the _____ is to blood.

3. Red blood cells are to carrying oxygen as _____ are to fighting germs.

4. Oxygen is to air as _____ are to food.

5. Carbon dioxide is to the circulatory system as _____ are to the digestive system.

6. Arteries are to carrying blood away from the heart as _____ are to carrying blood back to the heart.

7. A healthy diet is to controlling your weight as _____ is to building a strong heart and arteries.

8. The small intestine is to digested food as the _____ is to solid waste.

160

The Respiratory and Urinary Systems

Think About as You Read

- **How does your body take in oxygen?**
- **How do the kidneys clean the blood?**
- **How can diet and exercise help your systems?**

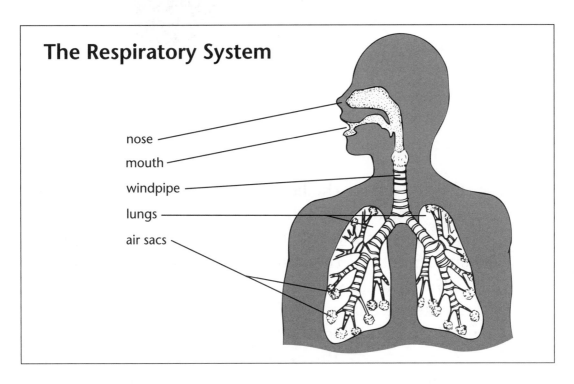

The Respiratory System

- nose
- mouth
- windpipe
- lungs
- air sacs

Your respiratory system is a group of organs that brings oxygen into your body.

Every cell in your body needs oxygen. It is the job of your **respiratory system** to bring oxygen into your body. As your blood carries nutrients and oxygen to the cells, wastes are formed. It is the job of your **urinary system** to clean your blood by removing liquid waste.

Your **respiratory system** takes in oxygen and gives off carbon dioxide.

How Does the Respiratory System Work?

Your respiratory system is the group of organs that brings oxygen into the body. This system also removes carbon dioxide waste from the body.

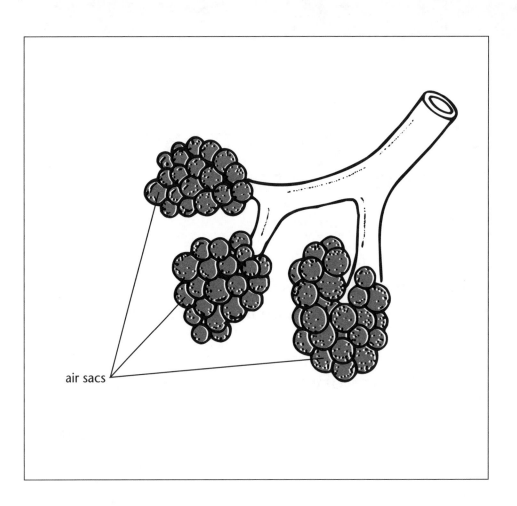

Millions of tiny air sacs are in your lungs. Oxygen in the air sacs goes into your blood.

Air sacs are tiny bags of air in the lungs that are surrounded by blood vessels.

Oxygen enters the body when you breathe in air. You can breathe air through your nose or your mouth. Your nose cleans and warms the air as you breathe. Your mouth cannot do this. So you should always try to breathe through your nose.

Air goes from the nose or mouth through a tube called the windpipe. Then air goes to the lungs.

Your lungs are the most important organ in the respiratory system. Millions of tiny **air sacs** are in the lungs. Tiny blood vessels surround each air sac. Oxygen from the air goes into the air sacs. The heart pumps blood to the lungs. Oxygen in the air sacs goes into the blood at the lungs. Then blood with oxygen leaves the lungs and goes back to the heart. Your heart pumps this blood to every part of the body.

You know that the veins carry blood with carbon dioxide waste back to the heart. The heart pumps this blood to the lungs. The blood gets rid of carbon dioxide in the lungs. Carbon dioxide leaves the lungs when you breathe out. Your respiratory system does this job thousands of times each day.

This is how the respiratory system works.

1. You breathe in air through the nose or mouth.
2. Air goes into the windpipe.
3. The windpipe carries air to the lungs.
4. In the lungs, oxygen from the air goes into the blood. Blood is pumped by the heart to all parts of the body.
5. Blood loses carbon dioxide in the lungs.
6. Carbon dioxide leaves the lungs when you breathe out air.

How to Care for Your Respiratory System

You should follow these six rules to take care of your respiratory system.

1. Do not smoke. Smoking causes lung disease.
2. Try to avoid breathing **polluted** air. Do not sit in areas of restaurants and airplanes that allow smoking. Avoid breathing dirty gases given off by cars, buses, and trucks.

Polluted describes something that is dirty and unhealthy.

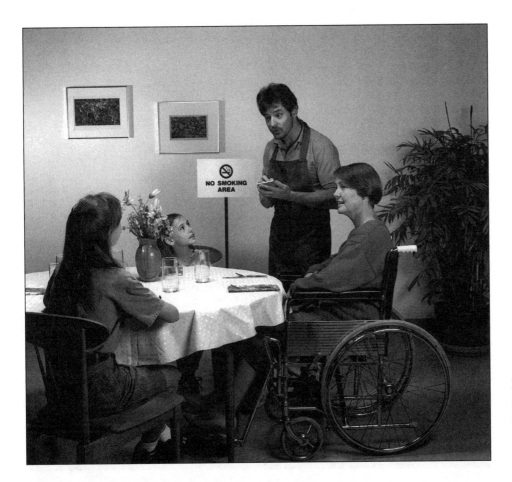

Many restaurants have areas that do not allow smoking.

163

3. Eat healthy foods and get enough sleep.
4. Exercise. Exercising makes your lungs strong.
5. See your doctor for regular checkups. Your doctor will listen to your lungs to make sure they are healthy.
6. Wear a face mask if you must be near dangerous gases or **asbestos**. You can badly damage your lungs by breathing dangerous gases or asbestos.

Asbestos is used to make a building material that does not burn. Asbestos was used in the ceilings or walls of older buildings.

Removing Wastes from the Body

Your body makes wastes as it uses nutrients and oxygen. The body must get rid of these wastes in order to be healthy. Your body has four ways to get rid of wastes.

1. You breathe out carbon dioxide waste from your lungs.
2. You remove **perspiration** through your skin when you sweat.
3. Your large intestine removes solid waste left by the foods you cannot digest.
4. Liquid waste is removed by the urinary system.

Perspiration is a liquid that is made by the body. It contains water, salt, and wastes from your blood.

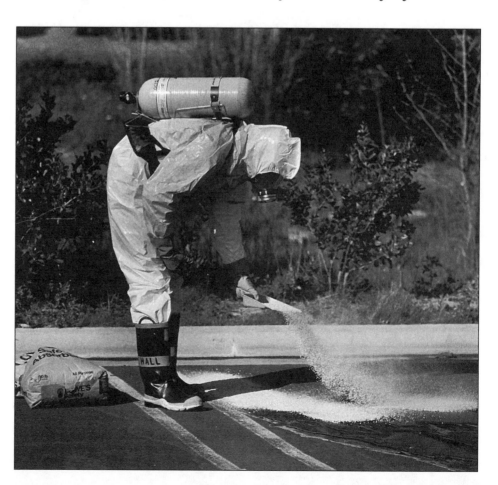

This firefighter wears a face mask and special clothes for protection from chemicals.

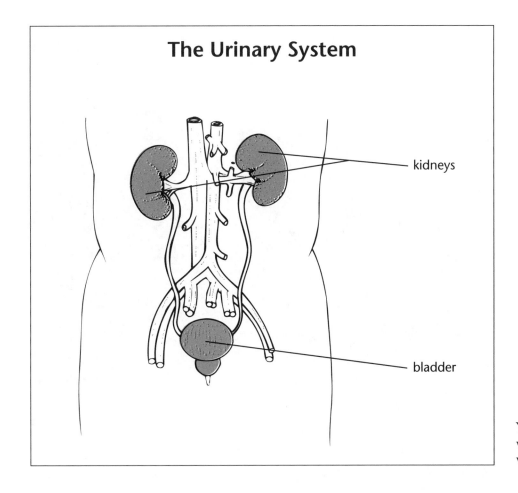

The Urinary System

Your kidneys make urine when they remove liquid waste from your blood.

The Urinary System

Your two **kidneys** are the most important part of the urinary system. The kidneys are in the lower back. Their job is to remove liquid waste from the blood. Kidneys make **urine** when they remove waste. Another organ, the **bladder**, holds the urine until you are ready to **urinate**.

Urine is the liquid waste that is made by the kidneys.

This is how the urinary system gets rid of waste.
1. Blood vessels carry blood to the kidneys.
2. Kidneys remove waste from the blood and make urine.
3. Urine leaves each kidney through a tube.
4. Each tube carries urine to the bladder.
5. The bladder holds urine.
6. Urine leaves the body when you urinate.

To **urinate** is to rid the body of urine.

Problems and Care of the Urinary System

Many people get bladder infections. You may have a bladder infection if you notice a painful or

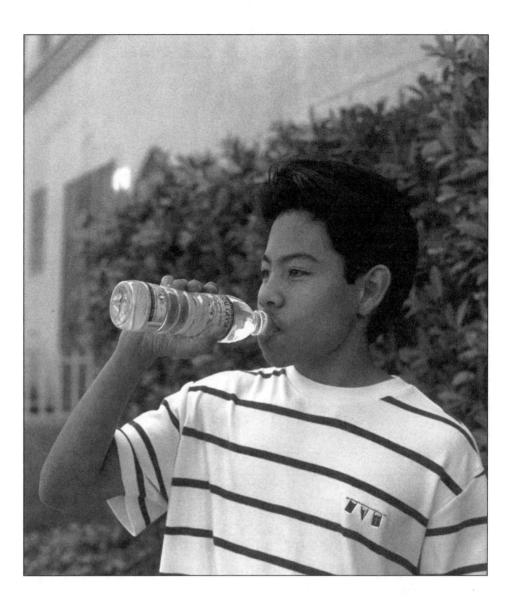

You can help keep your urinary system healthy by drinking six to eight glasses of water each day.

burning feeling when you urinate. You may notice a bad odor or see blood in your urine. You should see your doctor if you think you have an infection.

Kidney stones are another problem for some people. Small stones form in the kidneys and can cause pain. A doctor can treat and remove kidney stones.

You can keep your urinary system healthy by drinking six to eight glasses of water each day. See your doctor if you have a problem when you urinate. See your doctor if you have blood in your urine.

Your body must breathe in oxygen to be healthy. It must also breathe out carbon dioxide. Your urinary system must get rid of the liquid waste made by the body. Caring for your body's systems will help you have a healthy body.

Using What You Learned

Choose a word or words in the box to complete each sentence. Write the correct answers on your paper.

polluted	asbestos	respiratory system	Perspiration
bladder	Kidneys	air sacs	urinary system

1. There are millions of tiny _____ in the lungs.

2. Air that is _____ is dirty and unhealthy.

3. A _____ infection can make it painful to urinate.

4. Your _____ takes in oxygen and gives off carbon dioxide.

5. _____ make urine when they remove liquid waste from the body.

6. A building material called _____ can badly damage your lungs.

7. The _____ includes the kidneys and bladder.

8. _____ is a liquid that contains water, salt, and wastes from your blood.

Comprehension—Write the Questions

Below are the answers for some questions from this chapter. Read each answer. Then write on your paper a possible question to go with each answer. Use the question words to help you.

1. What _____ ?

   The urinary system's job is to clean the blood by removing liquid waste.

2. Where _____ ?

   Oxygen enters the body through the mouth and nose.

167

3. Who _____ ?

A doctor can treat and remove kidney stones.

4. What _____ ?

You should wear a face mask when working around dangerous gases or asbestos.

5. What _____ ?

The lungs are the most important organs in the respiratory system.

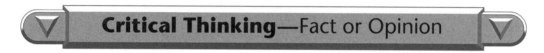

Critical Thinking—Fact or Opinion

Write **Fact** on your paper for each fact below. Write **Opinion** for each opinion. You should find three sentences that are opinions.

1. Drinking six to eight glasses of water each day can help keep your urinary system healthy.

2. Asbestos is harmful to the lungs.

3. Your respiratory system is the easiest system to keep healthy.

4. Smoking can cause lung disease.

5. Young people do not have to take care of their respiratory systems.

6. Small kidney stones can cause pain.

7. You might have a bladder infection if you have a painful feeling when you urinate.

8. Oxygen in the air sacs goes into the blood.

9. The windpipe carries air from the nose and mouth to the lungs.

10. The urinary system is more important than the respiratory system.

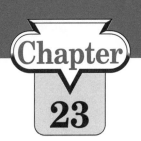

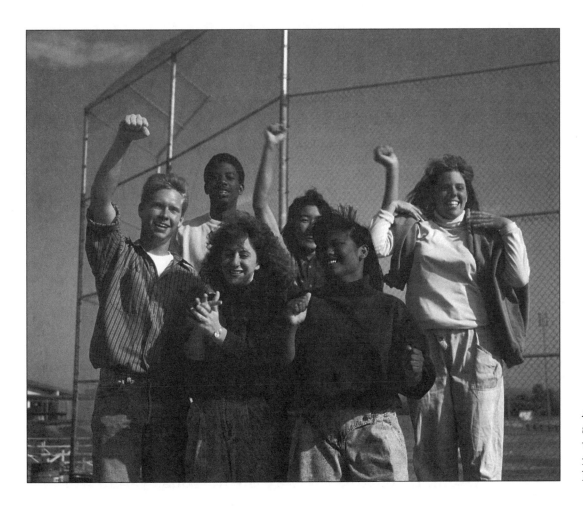

Chapter 23

Your Nervous and Endocrine Systems

Think About as You Read

- How does your brain help you think, walk, and breathe?
- Why does your body need hormones?
- How should you care for your body's systems?

All of your body systems must work together for you to be healthy.

The systems of your body perform important jobs. They digest food and get rid of wastes. They take in oxygen and get rid of carbon dioxide. Your body also has two systems that control the way all of the other systems work.

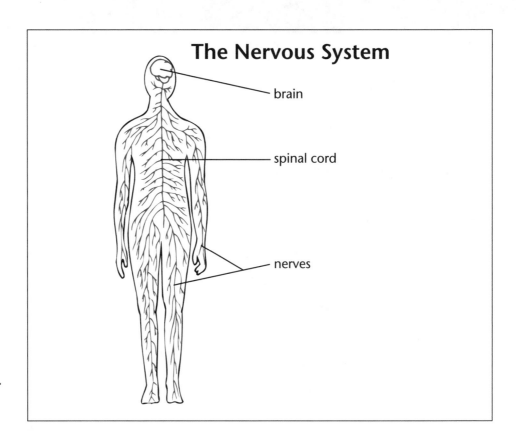

The Nervous System

Your nervous system controls your thinking, your heart, your breathing, and your movements.

Your **spinal cord** is a thick row of nerves that goes down the center of your back.

Thin, threadlike parts attached to nerve cells are nerve **fibers**.

The Nervous System

Your **nervous system** controls everything you do. It controls your thinking and learning. It controls the way your heart pumps and the way you move.

Your nervous system has three parts. The three parts are your brain, your **spinal cord**, and your nerves.

Your nervous system is made of nerve cells. Nerve cells carry messages to different parts of the body. Nerve cells have long **fibers.** The nerves in your body are groups of nerve fibers.

The Brain and Spinal Cord

Your brain is the most important part of the nervous system. It controls the way the nervous system works. The brain is made of nerve cells.

The brain has three parts. Each part of your brain does a different job.

1. The **cerebrum** controls your thinking, talking, and learning. You use your cerebrum when you do math, read, or spell.

2. The **cerebellum** controls the way your body moves. The cerebellum sends messages to your muscles so you can control the way you move. When you ride your bike, you are using your cerebellum.

3. The **medulla** controls your body's systems. It controls your breathing and the beating of your heart. It controls the work of the stomach and the small intestine. It controls the kidneys. Your medulla works even when you are asleep.

Your spinal cord is a thick group of nerves that goes down the center of your back. The spinal cord begins at your brain. It ends below your ribs. The spinal cord is protected by the bones of your spine. The nerves of the spinal cord are connected to nerves in all parts of your body. Nerves in different parts of the body are also connected to the spinal cord.

How does the nervous system work? Your brain sends messages through your nerves to all parts of your body. Nerves in different parts of your body send messages to the brain. These messages allow you to move. The messages also allow you to see, feel, smell, taste, and hear.

Taking Care of Your Nervous System

You should care for your nervous system by protecting your head and spinal cord. Always wear a helmet when you ride your bike or your skateboard.

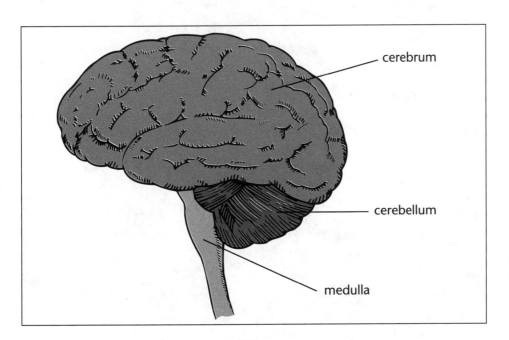

cerebrum

cerebellum

medulla

The most important part of the nervous system is the brain. It has three parts.

Protect your head when you swim. Many people hurt their heads in diving accidents. Never dive into water unless you know it is deep enough for diving.

Protect your head and spinal cord when riding in a car. Always wear a seat belt when riding in a car.

To care for your nervous system, you should get enough sleep. Do not use drugs incorrectly or alcohol. They can destroy the nerve cells of the brain.

Your Endocrine System

Your **endocrine system** has glands that make **hormones**. The glands send hormones into the blood. Your blood carries them to different parts of the body. Every hormone does a different job. Your body cannot work and grow properly without these hormones.

How do some of your glands help you? Your **pituitary gland** controls the way all of the other endocrine glands work. It also makes a growth hormone. This hormone controls the growth of your bones.

Your **endocrine system** makes chemicals that help your body work and grow properly.

Hormones are chemicals made by organs in the endocrine system to affect other parts of the body.

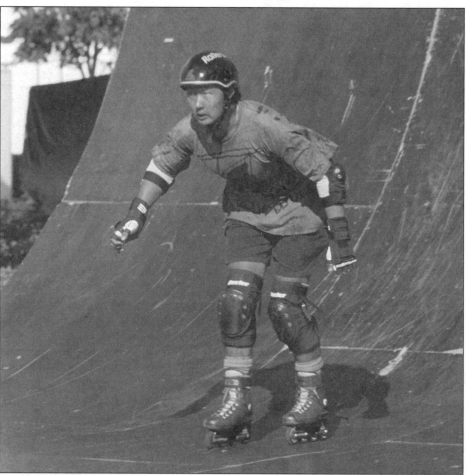

Wear a helmet whenever you need to protect your head.

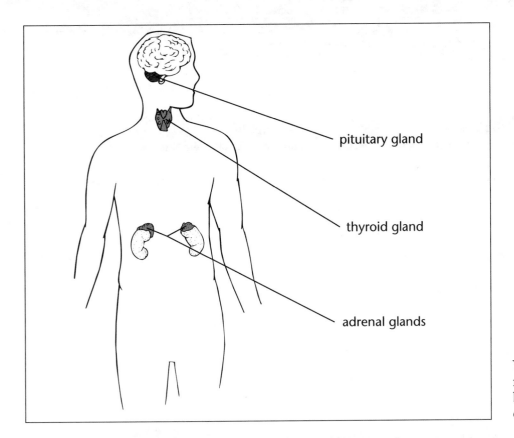

pituitary gland

thyroid gland

adrenal glands

Your endocrine system makes the hormones your body needs. Each hormone does a different job.

Your **adrenal glands** make adrenaline. This hormone helps your body deal with stress. When a person is very frightened, adrenaline makes the heart beat faster. Adrenaline makes people feel stronger and breathe faster.

Your **thyroid gland** makes a hormone that controls how fast your body uses food. Sometimes the thyroid gland does not make enough of this hormone. Then the body uses food slowly. This causes people to gain weight. The thyroid gland may make too much of this hormone. This can cause people to lose weight. A doctor can treat you if your thyroid gland makes too much or too little of this hormone.

Care for your endocrine system by taking care of your physical health. Eat healthy meals and get enough sleep. Try to exercise at least three times a week. Visit your doctor if you think you have a health problem.

You depend on your nervous and endocrine systems for good health. These two systems control the way your other body systems work for you.

Your **adrenal glands** make a hormone that helps the body handle fear and danger.

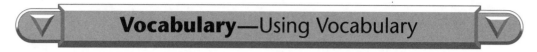
Vocabulary—Using Vocabulary

Use the word or words to write a complete sentence on your paper about your nervous or endocrine system.

1. nervous system
2. endocrine system
3. hormones
4. spinal cord
5. thyroid gland

Comprehension—Finish the Paragraph

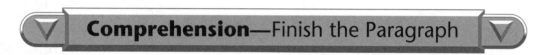

Number your paper from 1 to 8. Use a word or words from the box to finish each sentence. Write the correct answers on your paper.

messages	controls	brain	adrenal
pituitary	endocrine	glands	spinal cord

Your nervous system __(1)__ the way your body works. It is made up of your brain, your __(2)__ , and your nerves. Nerve cells in your __(3)__ control the way the nervous system works. Other nerve cells carry __(4)__ from your brain to different parts of your body.

Your __(5)__ system makes hormones that help your body work and grow properly. These hormones are made by __(6)__ . The __(7)__ glands make a hormone called adrenaline that helps your body deal with stress. Your __(8)__ gland controls all the other endocrine glands.

Comprehension—Writing About Health

Answer the following question in complete sentences on your paper.

What are three things you can do to care for your nervous system?

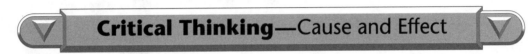 **Critical Thinking**—Cause and Effect

Write sentences on your paper by matching each cause on the left with an effect on the right.

Cause

1. Nerves in your ears and eyes send messages to your brain, so _____

2. Your medulla controls your body's systems, so _____

3. You are very frightened, so _____

4. Your cerebrum controls your thinking and learning, so _____

5. The cerebellum controls the way your body moves, so _____

6. You want to protect your nervous system, so _____

7. The thyroid gland does not make enough of its hormone, so _____

Effect

a. it makes you breathe and it makes your heart beat.

b. it helps you understand your math homework.

c. you are able to hear and see.

d. your adrenal glands release adrenaline.

e. you wear a helmet when riding your bike.

f. the body uses food slowly and gains weight.

g. it helps you swim and run.

UNIT 8

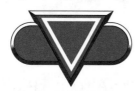

Family Health

Who are the people you really care about? You may care a lot about the members of your family or the family you live with. You may also care about your good friends.

To have good health, you must learn to make good decisions. You may learn these decision-making skills from your family or the family you live with. One day you may teach these skills to your own children.

Have You Ever Wondered?

▼ Our families meet many of our needs. Which needs?

▼ People see many changes in their bodies during the teen years. What kinds of changes?

▼ People who marry after the age of 22 often have better marriages. Why?

As you read this unit, think about things you can do to get along better with your family or the family you live with and your friends.

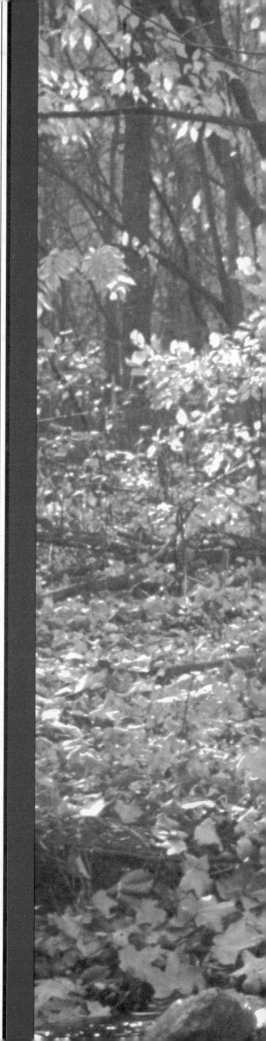

176

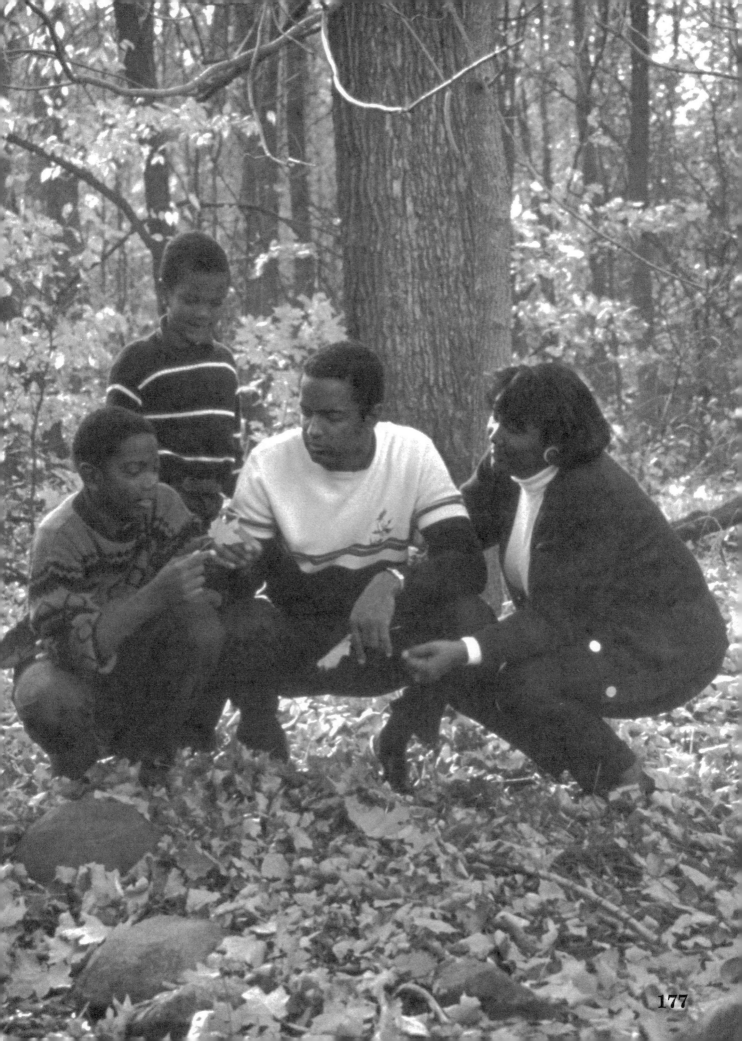

Living with Your Family

Think About as You Read

- **What are five different kinds of families?**
- **What kinds of problems do families have?**
- **How can you get along better with your family?**

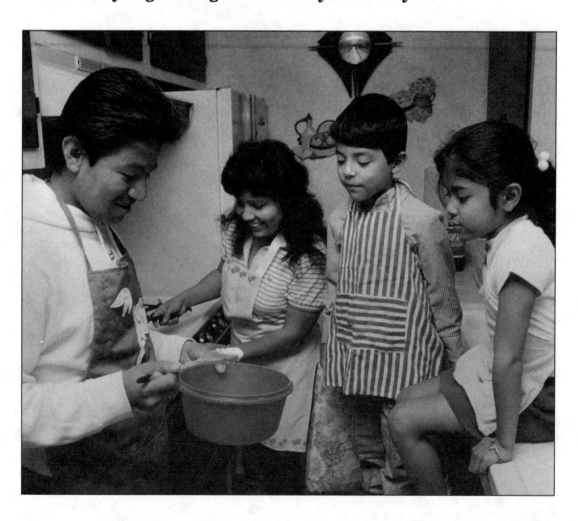

Family members enjoy doing things together.

You are a member of a family. Your family may share your good times and bad times.

Your family can help you in many ways. Getting along with the family you live with helps your physical health, social health, and emotional health.

Kinds of Families

Each family is different. Each family has its own rules and problems. Most families can tell stories about their special times together.

Here are five different kinds of families.

1. The **traditional family** has a mother and a father and one or more children.
2. The single-parent family has one parent and one or more children. Sometimes another adult who is not related to the family lives with the family.
3. A stepfamily has one **natural parent**, one stepparent, and one or more children. A stepparent is related to the family by marriage.

A **natural parent** is related to the child by blood.

4. An **extended family** has one or both parents, one or more children, and other family members living in a home.
5. A **foster family** has adults who take care of one or more children because the children's natural parents cannot care for them.

How Does Your Family Meet Your Needs?

Your family can meet your physical needs by giving you food and clothing. Your family also gives you a home in which to live.

In this extended family, the parents, the baby, and other family members live together.

Your family can meet your emotional needs by helping you feel love, acceptance, and success. You feel acceptance when you are loved even if you make mistakes or have problems. Your family gives you **responsibilities** to allow you to have success. You have high self-esteem when you know your family believes in you.

Your family also helps you learn **values**. The values in some families are to work hard, to have good manners, to be kind, and to be honest. Your values help you decide how to act.

Responsibilities are jobs you do that show you can be trusted to do things well.

Your **values** are your ideas about what is important.

Problems in Families

Every family has problems. Sometimes a parent loses a job. Sometimes a member of the family is very sick. Some families do not make enough money to buy the things they need. Drugs and alcohol cause terrible problems in some families.

Sometimes teen-agers have problems in a family. Their parents may not like their friends, their clothes, or their music.

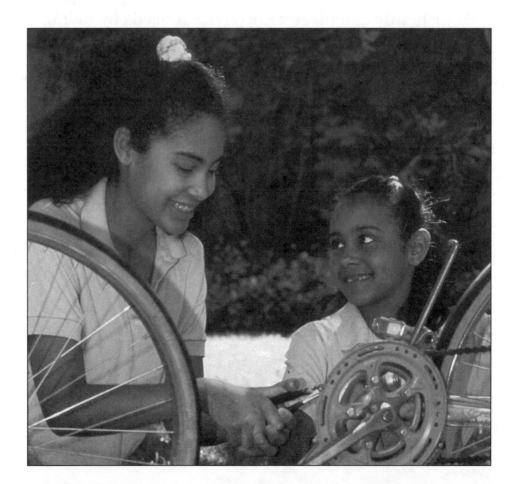

Your family can help you meet your emotional needs for love, acceptance, and success.

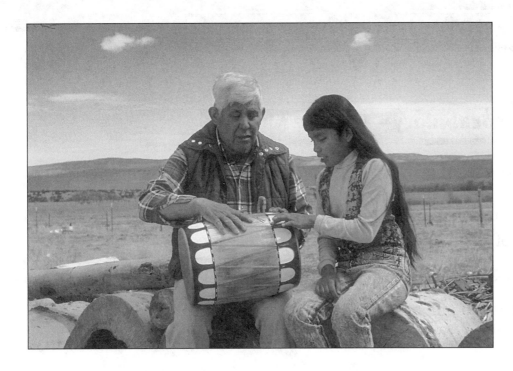

Work at getting along with your family. Speak with respect to family members. Be a good listener.

Leslie solved her family problem. She wanted to spend more time with her friends. Leslie told her mother and stepfather how she felt. Then she talked to them about how well she handled her responsibilities at home and at school. Leslie's parents decided to let her spend more time with her friends. They trusted her to make good decisions while she was with her friends.

Building a Strong Family

Talk to your family. Tell your family about the things that make you happy, sad, and angry. Speak with respect to family members. Be a good listener.

You can do five things to get along better with your family.

1. Do your share of jobs and chores at home.
2. Listen when family members talk about their problems and their successes.
3. Show respect for others.
4. Do things that you enjoy with your family.
5. Celebrate special holidays and birthdays with your family.

Learn to get along with your family. Then you will have the skills to get along with others when you are away from home.

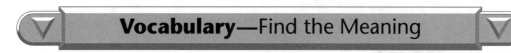

Using What You Learned

Write on your paper the word or words that best complete each sentence.

1. Adults who take care of children because the children's natural parents cannot take care of them are part of a _____ .

   traditional family   **extended family**   **foster family**

2. A mother, a father, and one or more children make up the _____ .

   good decisions   **traditional family**   **single-parent family**

3. The jobs you do that show you can be trusted to do things well are your _____ .

   responsibilities   **values**   **problems**

4. A _____ is the mother or father who is related to a child by blood.

   foster family   **stepparent**   **natural parent**

5. Your ideas about what is important are your _____ .

   friends   **chores**   **values**

Comprehension—Write the Questions

Below are the answers for some questions from this chapter. Read each answer. Then write on your paper a possible question to go with each answer. Use the question words to help you.

1. What _____ ?

   A single-parent family has one parent and one or more children.

2. Who _____ ?

   Your family helps you learn values.

3. Why _____?

   Your family gives you responsibilities to allow you to have success.

4. What _____?

   Your family meets your physical needs for food and clothing.

5. How _____?

   A stepparent is related to a family by marriage.

6. What _____?

   The values in some families are to work hard and to be honest.

7. What _____?

   Three ways you can get along better with your family are showing respect for them, talking with them, and doing your share of chores at home.

Critical Thinking—Analogies

Use a word or words in the box to finish each sentence. Write the correct answers on your paper.

emotional need	**self-esteem**	**stepfamily**
values	**extended family**	

1. Chores are to responsibilities as good manners and being honest are to _____.

2. Physical need is to food as _____ is to acceptance.

3. Responsibilities are to jobs as _____ is to good feelings.

4. Single-parent family is to one parent as _____ is to one natural parent and one stepparent.

5. Traditional family is to parents and children as _____ is to parents, children, and other family members.

Building Relationships

Think About as You Read

- Which communication skills can help you get along with others?
- How can you build strong friendships?
- Why should teen-agers say no to intimate sexual behavior?

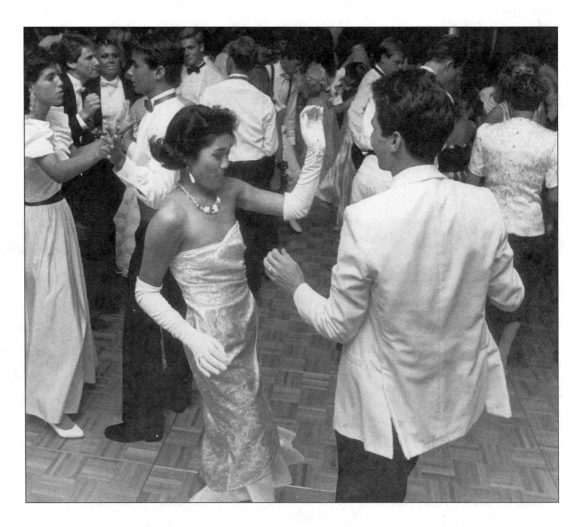

Boys and girls may start to form friendships with each other during the teen years.

Relationships are the way you get along with others.

Adam felt nervous at his first school dance. He had never danced with a girl. Building new **relationships** can be difficult. In this chapter you will read about ways to build relationships.

Improving Communication Skills

Share your ideas with others. This will help you build good relationships. These four communication skills can help you get along with others.

1. Be a good listener. Listen to what other people say. Then share your own ideas.
2. Do not talk about other people. People often find out what others say about them. People may be angry with you for talking about them.
3. Think carefully before you speak. Do not say things you may later feel sorry about. You may say the wrong things when you are angry or unhappy.
4. Use "I" messages when you talk about your feelings. Talk about how you think and feel instead of blaming others.

Different Kinds of Relationships

Every person needs love and friendship to have good emotional and social health. To have loving relationships, you must show people that you care.

Your first loving relationships are with your family. As you grow, you form other friendships. Every person needs friends.

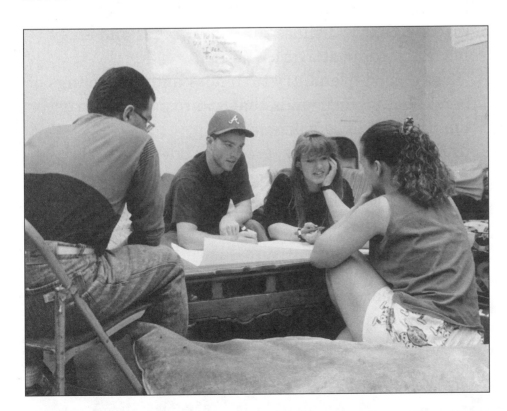

Learn how to share your ideas and feelings with others.

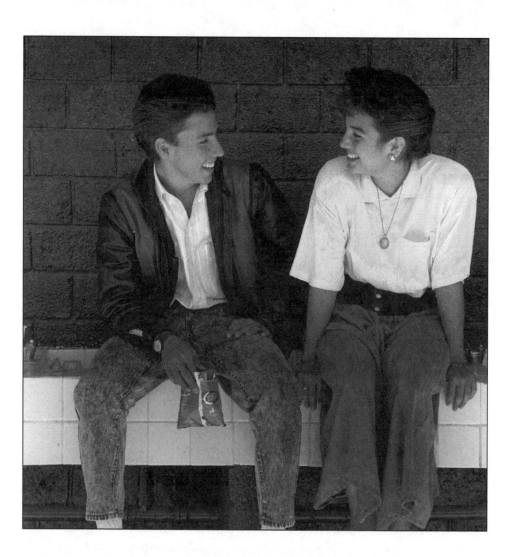

Choose your friends carefully. Show your friends that you care about them.

How can you build strong friendships? First, you must like yourself and accept yourself. Then others will like you, too. Choose your friends carefully. It is important that you share the same values and enjoy some of the same activities.

To be a good friend, try to understand the feelings of others. Show your friends that you respect and trust them. Be kind to your friends.

During the teen years, groups of boys and girls spend time together. They may go as a group to the movies or to a park. Some teens start to date.

Dating

Dating becomes important to some people during the early teen years. Other teens do not feel ready to date until they are older. Many parents make rules about the age when teens can start dating.

Some teens have low self-esteem if they do not have many dates. There are other ways teens can build self-esteem. Sharing activities and interests with friends builds self-esteem. Learning new skills also builds self-esteem.

How should you choose a person to date? You date a person you find attractive. The person should share your values. Your date should enjoy some of your interests. Your date should also have respect for you and your decisions.

You should show responsible behavior when you are on a date. Show good manners. Do not use alcohol or other drugs. Return home at the time your parents ask you to be home.

Sexual Behavior

All people have **sexual** feelings. Your sexual behavior is the way you show your sexual feelings.

Sexual behavior can be smiling at people of the **opposite sex** to show you like them. For some people sexual behavior can be holding hands, hugging, and kissing. Married adults have intimate sexual behavior.

Sexual describes anything that has to do with being a male or a female.

The **opposite sex** is the one that is different from your own. If you are a male, a member of the opposite sex is a female.

Holding hands is one kind of sexual behavior. You should avoid high-risk sexual behavior.

187

You may feel pressure to have intimate sexual behavior when dating. As a teen-ager you are making a wise decision when you say no to intimate sexual behavior. Here are three reasons for a teen-ager to say no.

1. You can get **AIDS** and other **sexually transmitted diseases** through intimate sexual behavior. AIDS is a terrible disease that kills people.

2. Intimate sexual behavior can lead to **pregnancy**.

3. Intimate sexual behavior can cause stress. You can feel guilty. You may worry about pregnancy. You may also worry about getting AIDS and other diseases. Your date may want you to have intimate sexual behavior again. Other people may learn about your intimate sexual behavior from your date.

Decide before a date what type of sexual behavior is right for you. It is healthy and safe to choose **abstinence**. Try hard to avoid risk behaviors.

The chart below shows three problems you may worry about when you say no to intimate sexual behavior. The chart also gives you answers for these problems. Never let your date talk you into doing something that you do not want to do.

Every person needs love and friendship. Your relationships can help you reach your goal of wellness.

AIDS is a disease in which the body cannot fight germs. AIDS can be spread through body liquids. There is no cure for AIDS.

Sexually transmitted diseases are diseases that can be spread from person to person through intimate sexual behavior.

Pregnancy is having one or more unborn children growing inside a female's body.

Abstinence is choosing not to do something. People may choose not to have intimate sexual behavior.

Dating and Sexual Behavior

Problem:	*Answer:*
1. My date may not want to see me again if I choose abstinence.	1. Your date should enjoy your company without intimate sexual behavior.
2. My friends will laugh at me if they learn I choose abstinence.	2. A real friend never wants you to hurt yourself with a risk behavior.
3. No one will want to date me if I choose abstinence.	3. Other people also choose abstinence. They will want to date you. They will approve of your decision.

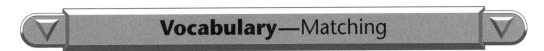

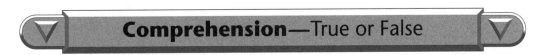

Vocabulary—Matching

Match each vocabulary word in **Group B** with a sentence from **Group A** that tells about the word. Write the letter of the correct answer on your paper.

Group A

1. This means choosing not to do something.

2. This is a disease in which the body cannot fight germs.

3. These can be spread through intimate sexual behavior.

4. This is having an unborn child growing inside a female's body.

5. You use good communication skills to build these.

Group B

a. AIDS

b. relationships

c. abstinence

d. pregnancy

e. sexually transmitted diseases

Comprehension—True or False

Write **True** on your paper for each sentence that is true. Write **False** on your paper for each sentence that is false. There are three false sentences. Rewrite the false sentences on your paper to make them true.

1. Being a good listener can help you get along with others.

2. Only adults have sexual feelings.

3. AIDS can be spread through intimate sexual behavior.

4. Sharing activities and interests with friends lowers self-esteem.

5. Abstinence can lead to sexually transmitted diseases.

189

6. Every person needs friends.

7. Intimate sexual behavior can cause stress.

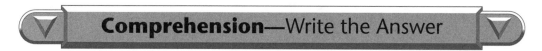

Comprehension—Write the Answer

Write a sentence on your paper to answer each question.

1. What kind of communication skills can help you get along with others?

2. What does every person need to have good emotional and social health?

3. What are three ways to be a good friend?

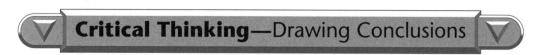

Critical Thinking—Drawing Conclusions

Read the paragraph. Then use the six steps below to decide what to do about building new relationships. Write complete sentences on your paper to answer each question.

> Imagine that in your class there is a new student who is of the opposite sex. You enjoy doing healthy activities after school with this new student. But your other friends are angry because you don't spend as much time with them.

Step 1. What is the problem?

Step 2. What are two ways to solve the problem?

Step 3. What is one consequence for each choice listed in Step 2?

Step 4. Which choice do you think is best?

Step 5. What can you do to put your decision into action?

Step 6. Think about your decision. Why was this the best choice for you?

Growth During the Teen Years

Think About as You Read

- How do males change during puberty?
- How do females change during puberty?
- What emotional and social changes take place during the teen years?

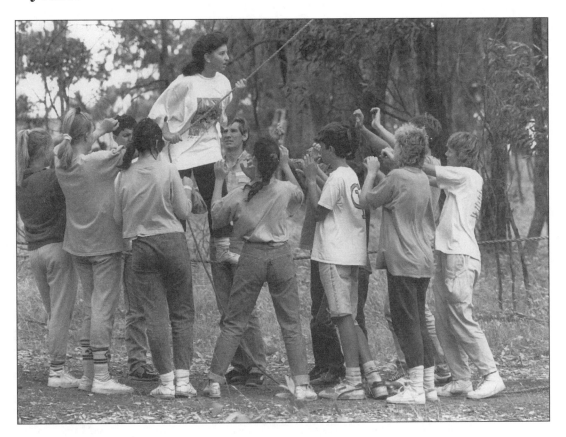

During the teen years, your body changes. You will have social and emotional changes, too.

Fourteen-year-old Pablo has more hair on his face than he did last year. His body has changed in other ways since he was 13. He has grown taller. He has gained weight. He has more hair on his body. Pablo is going through the changes of **puberty**. In this chapter you will learn how males and females change during puberty.

Puberty is the time when the sex organs and the sex glands begin to work.

Understanding Puberty

Reproductive organs are the parts of the body that allow males and females to produce children.

Mature describes something or someone that is fully grown or fully developed.

Every person is born with **reproductive organs**. In order for a male and a female to have a baby, their reproductive organs must **mature**. The reproductive organs slowly mature during puberty.

Many changes take place in your body at puberty. You grow taller. You gain weight faster. More hair grows on your body. Oil glands and sweat glands work much harder. Your skin and hair may be more oily. You may have pimples and blackheads. You may need to wash your hair more often.

Puberty is different for each person. Puberty affects males and females differently.

Some people go through puberty in the early teen years. For others puberty starts later. Some people grow and develop much faster than others. For others puberty lasts longer. By the end of puberty, every person's body has matured into the body of an adult.

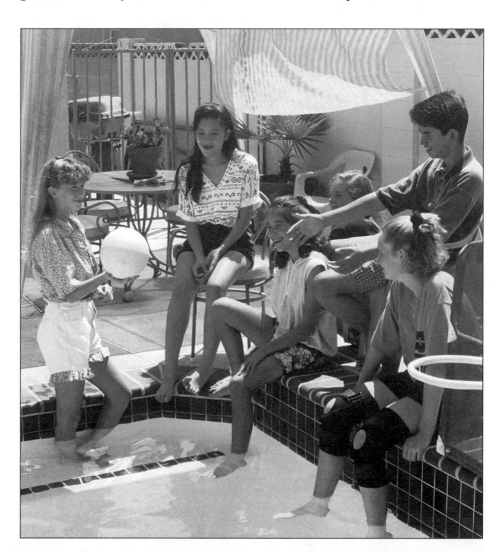

Puberty is different for each person. By the end of puberty, every person has a mature body.

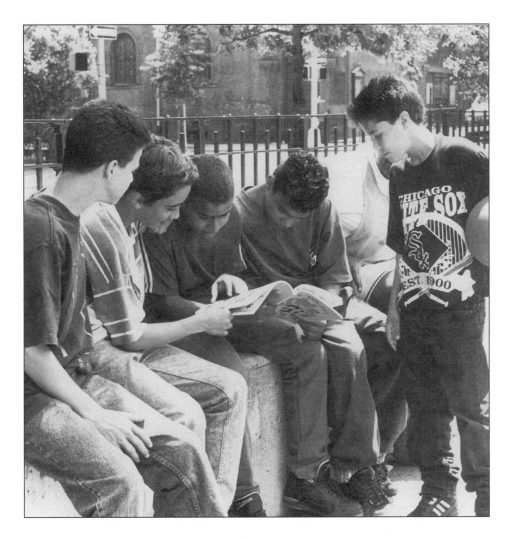

Hormones cause the changes of puberty. Males and females have different sex hormones.

Hormones cause all of the changes during puberty. You have learned that the endocrine glands make hormones. The pituitary gland sends hormones into the blood during puberty. These hormones make your bones grow. They make your sex glands start to work. Then the sex glands make their own hormones.

Males and Puberty

During puberty a male's **testes** start to produce male sex hormones. These hormones cause hair to grow on a male's face and chest. They cause a male's voice to become deeper. The male sex hormones cause his shoulders to become wider.

The **testes** are the male endocrine glands that make male sex hormones.

Male hormones make the male sex organs mature. The testes start to produce **sperm cells**. When a sperm cell from a male enters an egg cell inside a female, she becomes pregnant.

Sperm cells are male reproductive cells.

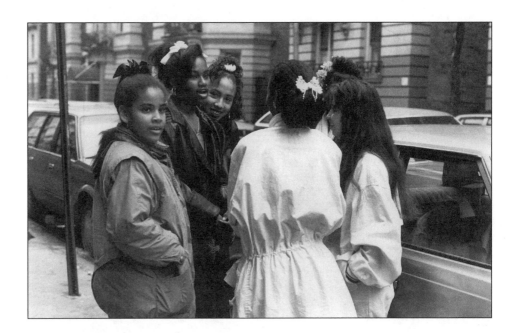

During puberty the ovaries start to make female hormones.

Ovaries are female sex glands that produce female hormones and egg cells.

Menstruation is the three-to-seven-day period when the egg cell flows out of the uterus with some blood.

The **uterus** is the female organ where a developing baby grows during pregnancy.

Females and Puberty

A female has two **ovaries**. The ovaries have thousands of tiny egg cells. During puberty the ovaries start to make female hormones. These hormones make a female's breasts grow larger. Her hips grow wider. The egg cells in the ovaries mature.

Menstruation also begins during puberty. Most females begin menstruation at about age 12. About every 28 days, an egg cell leaves one of the ovaries. It travels through one of the two **Fallopian tubes** to the **uterus**. Menstruation starts about two weeks after an egg cell leaves the ovary. Menstruation starts if a female is not pregnant. During menstruation the egg cell flows out of the uterus with some blood. This flow is also called a "period." The flow of blood lasts between three and seven days.

A female may have a period about every 28 days. Some females may have a period every 25 days or every 35 days. Sometimes it takes a few years for a female's period to become regular. Then she will usually have her period around the same time each month.

Many females have questions about their periods. They should ask their parents, doctor, or school nurse any questions they have.

194

Emotional and Social Changes During Puberty

Many teen-agers have low self-esteem during puberty. They may feel unhappy with their changing bodies. Some teen-agers mature earlier than their friends. These teens may think they look too grown-up. Other teen-agers mature later than their friends. These teens may have low self-esteem because they look less grown-up than their friends.

Teen-agers want more freedom and responsibility as they grow older. They may want to hold a job and drive a car. Teens often want more freedom from their parents. They want to spend more time with friends and less time with their family. Many teens no longer like the same music, dances, or clothes that their parents enjoy. Spending time alone can be important to teen-agers.

Many teens start dating. They must think about having responsible sexual behavior. They must avoid risk behaviors when dating.

Every person must go through the changes of puberty. By making responsible decisions, teens can reach the goal of wellness.

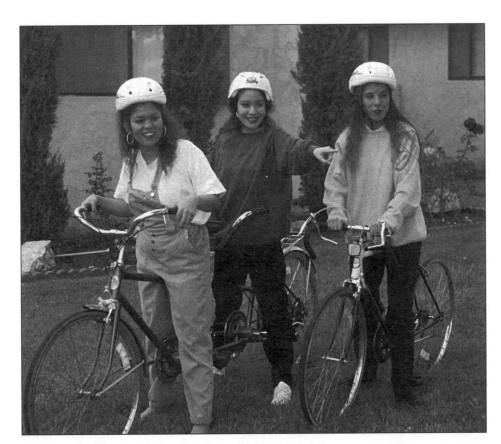

Many teen-agers want to spend more time with their friends and less time with their parents.

Using What You Learned

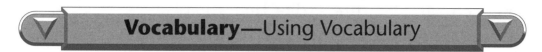

Vocabulary—Using Vocabulary

Use each word to write a complete sentence on your paper about growth during the teen years.

1. puberty
2. mature
3. menstruation
4. hormones
5. testes
6. ovaries

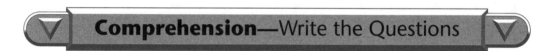

Comprehension—Write the Questions

Below are the answers for some questions from this chapter. Read each answer. Then write on your paper a possible question to go with each answer. Use the question words to help you.

1. What _____ ?

   Puberty is the time when the sex organs and the sex glands begin to work.

2. When _____ ?

   Many changes take place in the body at puberty.

3. Where _____ ?

   An egg cell travels through one of the two Fallopian tubes to the uterus.

4. When _____ ?

   Menstruation starts about two weeks after an egg cell leaves the ovary.

Comprehension—Finish the Paragraph

Number your paper from 1 to 8. Use a word from the box to finish each sentence. Write the correct answers on your paper.

glands	hair	taller	different
organs	deeper	hormones	wider

During the teen years, you and your friends grow and develop at __(1)__ rates. All of the changes of puberty are caused by __(2)__. Hormones help you to grow __(3)__. They make more __(4)__ grow on your body. Hormones make your oil and sweat __(5)__ work harder. They also cause your reproductive __(6)__ to mature. Male hormones make a male's voice __(7)__. Female hormones make a female's hips grow __(8)__.

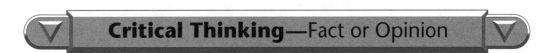

Critical Thinking—Fact or Opinion

Write **Fact** on your paper for each fact. Write **Opinion** for each opinion. You should find three sentences that are opinions.

1. It is easier for boys to go through puberty than it is for girls.

2. Every person is born with reproductive organs.

3. Menstruation takes place only if the female is not pregnant.

4. Every person goes through many changes during puberty.

5. Making responsible decisions is always easy.

6. You should never spend time alone during puberty.

7. Many teen-agers want to spend more time with their friends than with their family.

Chapter 27

The Life Cycle

Think About as You Read

- How should a female care for her unborn baby?
- What are the five stages of the life cycle?
- What makes each person different from every other person?

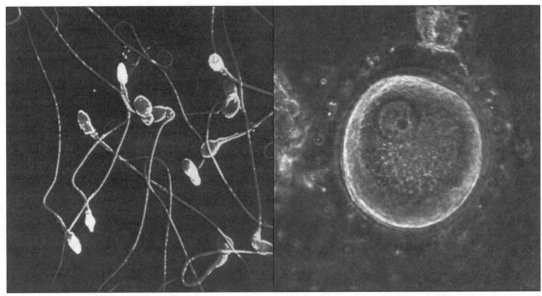

A new life begins when a sperm cell from a male joins an egg cell from a female.

sperm cells   egg cell

The **life cycle** is the five stages of life from birth until death.

Every person begins life as one cell that grows into a baby. People go through different stages of the **life cycle**. At the end of the life cycle, all living things die.

A New Life Begins

A new life begins when a sperm cell from a male joins an egg cell from a female. The two cells join in one of the female's Fallopian tubes. When the sperm cell and the egg cell join, they form a **fertilized egg**. The female becomes pregnant. This fertilized egg can grow into a baby.

The fertilized egg travels from the Fallopian tube into the uterus. Inside the uterus it grows into a baby. First, the fertilized egg divides into two cells. Then these cells divide again and again. Soon there are millions of cells. The cells begin to form organs. By the end of one month, the baby has a tiny beating heart.

The growing baby gets its nutrients and oxygen through an **umbilical cord**. This cord attaches the mother's uterus and the baby's navel. Nutrients and oxygen from the mother's body go through the blood vessels in the umbilical cord to the baby.

A pregnancy should last about nine months. At the end of that time, the baby is ready to be born.

The birth of a baby begins with **labor**. During labor the muscles of the female's uterus push the baby down towards the **vagina**. At birth the baby comes out of the mother's vagina. The head should come out first. The umbilical cord is cut right after birth.

The **umbilical cord** is a thick cord made of blood vessels that connects the baby's navel to its mother's uterus.

Labor is the physical work done by a female's body to give birth to a baby.

The **vagina** is the part of a female's body that goes from the uterus to outside the body.

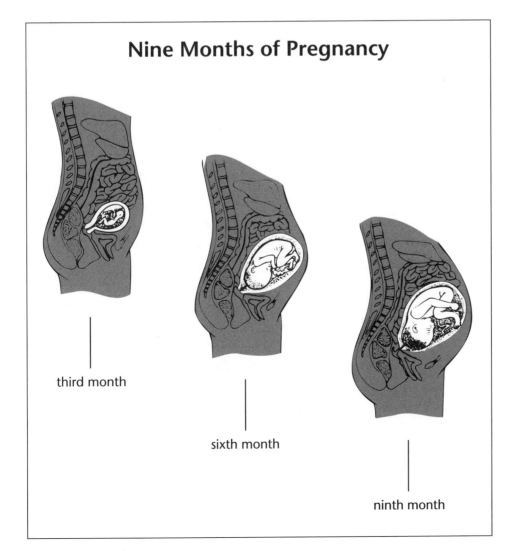

Nine Months of Pregnancy

third month

sixth month

ninth month

A baby should grow in its mother's uterus for nine months.

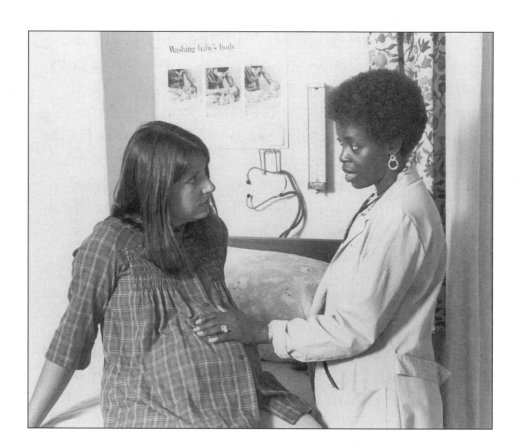

There are many things a pregnant female should do to have a healthy baby.

Sometimes the baby cannot be born by passing through the vagina. Doing so may be dangerous for the mother or for the baby. If there is a problem, the female may have an operation called a **Cesarean section** to have the baby.

Caring for the Unborn Baby

To have a healthy baby, a pregnant female should take care of herself in these six ways.

1. See a doctor as often as necessary for checkups.
2. Eat a healthy diet. A pregnant female must get enough nutrients. She needs extra calcium and iron in her diet.
3. Get enough sleep and rest.
4. Never use drugs in ways that are not correct. Do not drink alcohol. Drugs and alcohol can damage the new baby's brain and body.
5. Do not smoke. The babies of smoking mothers are often smaller and less healthy.
6. Do not take any medicine without checking with a doctor.

The Life Cycle

There are five stages in the human life cycle.

1. The nine months of pregnancy are the first stage of the life cycle.

2. Childhood is the time from birth to the teen years. The new baby grows. It learns to sit, walk, and talk. During this stage the child is always learning new skills.

3. During the teen years, the teen-ager grows into an adult. By the age of 19, many teens have reached their full height. They develop new skills. Friendships are especially important.

4. The adult years are from age 20 to about age 65. To have a strong, healthy body, an adult must exercise and have healthy eating habits. Adults may get married and have children. Emotional and social growth continues during the adult years.

5. Older adults are age 65 or older. Many older adults continue to play sports and exercise. They may retire from their jobs. Then they may spend more time doing hobbies. Older adults may develop health problems. This stage of the life cycle ends when the person dies.

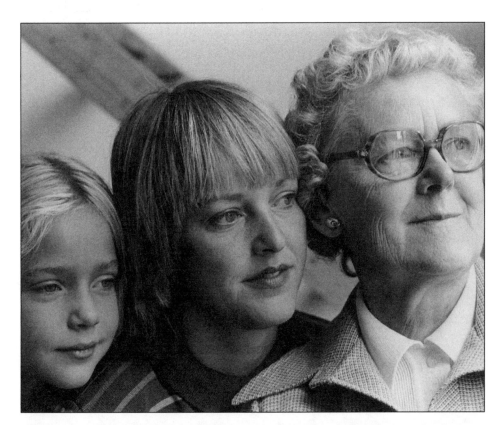

Childhood, adult years, and older adult years are three stages of the life cycle.

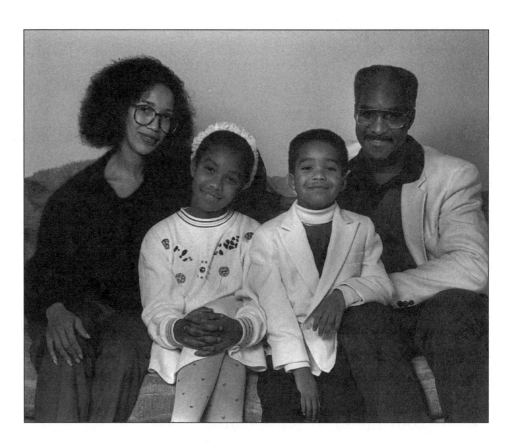

You inherit many traits from both parents. Some traits are for skin, hair, and eye color.

Each Person Is Different

As you go through the life cycle, many things about you change. The way you look, think, act, or feel may change. Let's look at what makes you special.

You are different from every other person. You were born with your own group of **traits**. Some of your traits have to do with how you look. These traits include your hair color, your skin color, your eye color, and your height. Other traits have to do with the way you act, think, and feel.

You **inherited** many traits from your parents. The egg cell from your mother and the sperm cell from your father each carried information about traits. You know that the sperm and egg joined to form a fertilized egg. This fertilized egg carried traits from both parents.

The kind of person you are begins with inherited traits. But the kind of person you become depends on what happens to you in your **environment**. Your home, family, friends, and your school are part of your environment. Your environment can affect what you learn. It may also affect the skills you have.

Traits are characteristics, such as skin and eye color, that belong to each person.

Inherited means a person received certain traits from his or her parents.

The **environment** includes the people, places, and objects that are around a person.

Your family environment makes you different from someone else. Maybe you are the oldest child in the family. You may have the responsibility of taking care of your younger brothers and sisters. If you are the youngest child in a family, you may not have this kind of responsibility. If you have lived in different cities, you may have had different experiences than people who have lived in the same city or town all their lives.

Your environment affects your traits. Try to use your environment to improve your traits. You may have a trait for curly or straight hair. You can learn to take care of your hair so it is clean and healthy.

People are born with many good traits. Use your traits to have success and good health. To do this you should make wise decisions during every stage of the life cycle. Try to make decisions that will help you reach the goal of wellness.

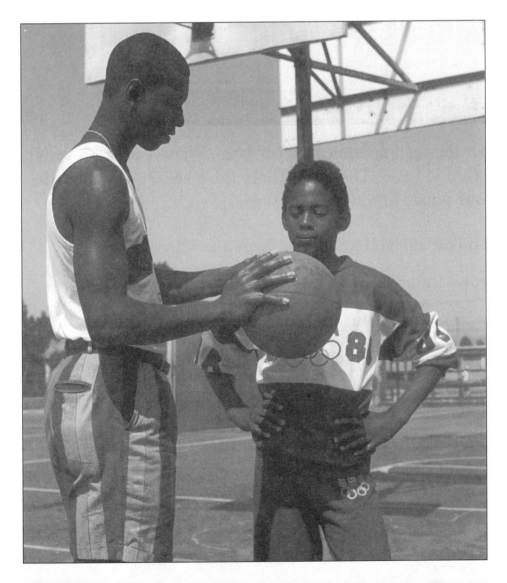

You may have traits that allow you to be good at sports. Work at improving your traits.

Using What You Learned

Vocabulary—Finish the Sentence

Choose a word or words in the box to complete each sentence. Write the correct answers on your paper.

| life cycle   umbilical cord   inherit   labor   environment |

1. A baby's navel is attached to the mother's uterus by an _____ .

2. The characteristics you _____ from your parents are called traits.

3. The people, places, and objects around you are part of your _____ .

4. The human _____ has five stages.

5. The birth of a baby begins with _____ .

Comprehension—True or False

Write **True** on your paper for each sentence that is true. Write **False** on your paper for each sentence that is false. There are three false sentences. Rewrite the false sentences on your paper to make them true.

1. When a sperm cell and an egg cell join, they form a fertilized egg.

2. The fertilized egg grows into a baby in the Fallopian tube.

3. A normal pregnancy lasts about four months.

4. At birth the baby comes out of the mother's vagina.

5. The first stage of the life cycle is the nine months of pregnancy.

6. You inherit many traits from both parents.

7. Your environment has no effect on the kind of person you are.

204

Comprehension—Writing About Health

Answer the following question in complete sentences on your paper.

What are three things a pregnant female can do for her unborn baby?

 Critical Thinking—Cause and Effect

Write sentences on your paper by matching each cause on the left with an effect on the right.

Cause

1. A pregnant female wants to have a healthy baby, so _____

2. A sperm cell from the male joins an egg cell from the female, so _____

3. The muscles of the uterus push down on the baby, so _____

4. The umbilical cord connects the baby's navel to the mother's uterus, so _____

5. You are the oldest child in your family, so _____

6. You make wise decisions throughout your life, so _____

Effect

a. the baby gets nutrients and oxygen from its mother.

b. the baby is born.

c. she takes good care of herself.

d. the female becomes pregnant.

e. you have success and good health.

f. your parents depend on you to do certain chores.

Marriage and Parenthood

Think About as You Read

- **What are the right and wrong reasons to get married?**
- **Why are teen-agers too young to be parents?**
- **How should parents care for their children?**

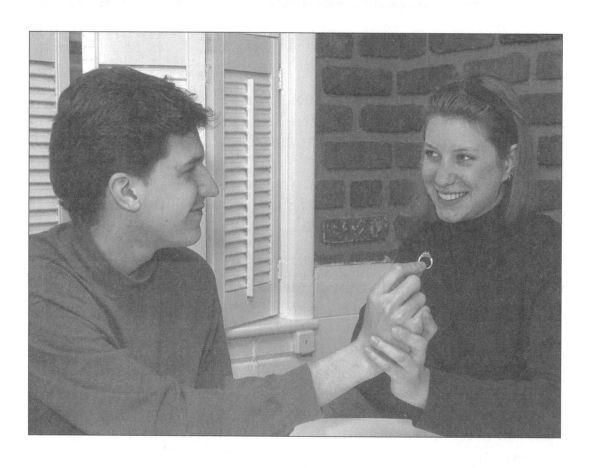

People who get married for the right reasons can be happy together.

Jennifer has been dating Rick for two years. Rick is 17. Jennifer is 16. Jennifer does not get along with her parents. She wants to drop out of school, get a job, and marry Rick. Rick says he is not ready to get married. What do you think Jennifer and Rick should do? In this chapter you will learn how couples can build good marriages and happy families.

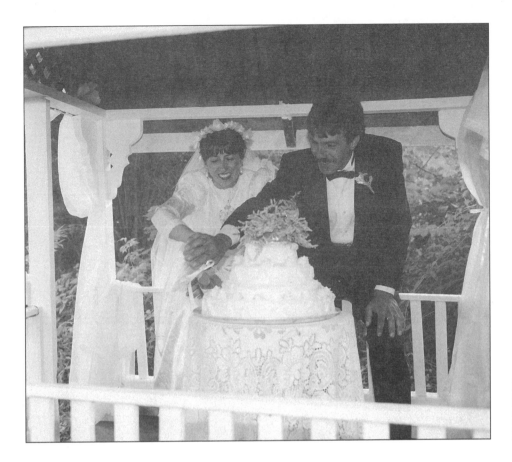

People who marry should love and care for each other. They should share important values.

Why Do People Get Married?

There are three very good reasons for a couple to get married. First, the couple shares interests and values. They enjoy being together. Second, they love and care for each other. Third, the couple communicates with each other. They share their feelings and solve problems.

Let's look at four of the wrong reasons people get married.

1. A couple gets married because of family pressure. Their parents want them to get married.
2. People get married because of peer pressure. Most of their friends are getting married.
3. A couple gets married because the female becomes pregnant.
4. Some people get married because they have an unhappy home life. They are unhappy living with their parents, brothers, and sisters. These people get married to escape family problems.

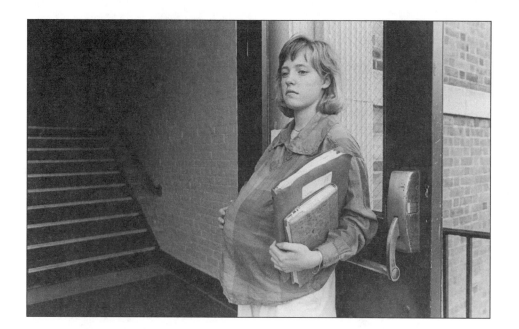

Teen-age mothers have problems. It is hard for them to finish high school and get good jobs.

Teen-age Marriages

Many teens marry because of peer pressure or to escape an unhappy home life. Many teen couples marry because the female is pregnant. Teen-agers often are not ready for family responsibilities.

Most teen marriages are unhappy. Married teen-agers often drop out of high school. Because they have not completed their education, they cannot get good jobs. They cannot earn enough money to buy the things they want or need. Most married teens do not understand the problems and feelings of the other person. They do not enjoy taking care of a home, washing clothes, and cooking meals every day. They want more time to have fun.

Many babies are born to teen-age females who are not married. Teen-age mothers and their babies have many problems. It is hard for teen-age mothers to finish high school and get good jobs. Taking care of their babies keeps teens so busy they have little time for fun. Some teen mothers may become **child abusers.** These teen mothers hurt their children because they are unhappy caring for the children.

Child abusers are people who hurt children in ways that are not accidents.

Teen-age females should avoid becoming pregnant. They should say no to intimate sexual behavior. They should choose abstinence.

208

Happy and Unhappy Marriages

To have a happy marriage, a couple should be mature. Most people who get married after the age of 22 have a better chance at having a happy marriage. People have better marriages when they share goals. Their goals may be to buy a house or have children. Couples must want to share good times and bad times together. They must trust each other. Earning enough money to pay for the things a couple wants and needs also helps a marriage.

Communication helps a marriage. People must share ideas and feelings. Couples should solve problems together. The husband and wife must learn to **compromise**.

Many marriages are not happy. Each year more than one million marriages end in divorce. Couples divorce for many different reasons. Divorce may be the last step for couples who have tried to work things out and to improve their marriage.

To **compromise** means to reach an agreement by having each side give up part of its demands.

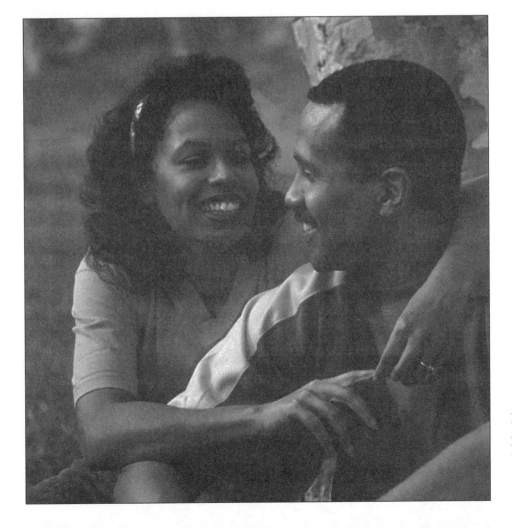

Happy couples share ideas and solve problems. They learn how to compromise.

A couple must go to court to get a divorce. A judge must decide whether to allow the couple to divorce. The judge also decides how the divorced couple will divide money and property from their marriage. The judge decides the best way to take care of any children the couple may have.

Most divorced people get married again. They often marry people who have children from another marriage. New stepfamilies are formed.

Counseling can help divorced families. It helps them talk about their feelings. Counseling helps them live with their new families and stepfamilies.

Counseling is giving advice and sharing ideas in order to help people solve their problems.

Becoming Parents

Many married couples want to have children. Couples should plan when to have children. They should talk about how many children they want.

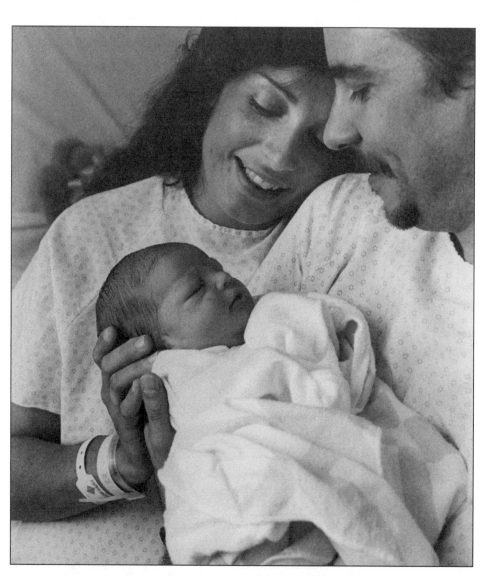

Many married couples want to have children.

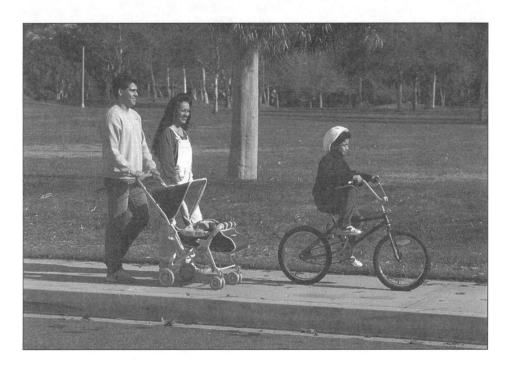

Parents can help their children have good emotional, physical, and social health.

Children need love, food, and clothes. They need a good home and medical care. They need time and attention from their parents. Parents must be able to take care of their children's needs. Parents need enough money to pay for things their children need.

Many children live in homes with only one parent. The single parent must do the work of both the mother and father. It is a hard job. But many single parents do a fine job.

Parents want their children to have good physical, social, and emotional health. Here are six things parents can do to help their children have wellness.

1. Parents can help their children set goals that can be reached.
2. They can show their children they love them.
3. Parents can teach values to their children.
4. They can teach their children correct behavior.
5. Parents can share ideas and feelings with their children.
6. They can teach their children decision-making skills.

Married people must work hard to have a good marriage and a happy family. Family life helps people have good physical, social, and emotional health.

Using What You Learned

Vocabulary—Matching

Match each vocabulary word in **Group B** with a sentence from **Group A** that tells about the word. Write the letter of the correct answer on your paper.

Group A

1. To have a happy marriage, a couple should be this.

2. A person who hurts a child in a way that is not an accident is called this.

3. People may need this in order to solve their problems.

4. Two people give up some of their demands to reach this agreement.

5. Teen-age females should choose this to avoid becoming pregnant.

Group B

a. abstinence

b. compromise

c. child abuser

d. mature

e. counseling

Comprehension—Write the Answer

Write a sentence on your paper to answer each question.

1. How does peer pressure make people want to get married?

2. Why does communication help a marriage?

3. Who decides the best way to take care of the children of a divorced couple?

4. What kinds of problems do married teen-agers have?

5. How can teen-age females avoid getting pregnant?

6. Why do some divorced families go to counseling?

Write **Fact** on your paper for each fact below. Write **Opinion** for each opinion. You should find three sentences that are opinions.

1. Sharing interests and values is the best reason to get married.
2. Communication can lead to a happy marriage.
3. Teen-agers often are not ready for family responsibilities.
4. Divorced people should not get married again.
5. A single parent cannot take good care of his or her children.
6. Some people get married because of family or peer pressure.
7. Counseling can help divorced parents talk about their feelings.

 Critical Thinking—Categories

Read the words in each group. Decide how they are alike. Find the best title in the box for each group. Write the title on your paper.

Wrong Reasons to Marry	Parents' Responsibilities
Divorce	Good Reasons to Marry

1. share interests and values
   love and care for each other
   communicate well

2. marriage problems
   end an unhappy marriage
   money and property divided

3. unhappy home life
   female gets pregnant
   peer pressure

4. show their children love
   teach their children values
   take care of their children's needs

UNIT 9

▽

Drug Abuse

Young people across the nation are doing important work. They have formed groups to teach each other to say no to drugs.

Would you want to hurt your family, lose good friends, and destroy your health? Of course you wouldn't. But millions of drug abusers hurt themselves and others each year. You can protect yourself by learning about drugs. Learn how drugs harm your physical, emotional, and social health. Then learn to say no to peer pressure and to avoid risk behaviors.

Have You Ever Wondered?

▼ It is dangerous to try drugs or drink alcohol even once. Why?

▼ There is one illegal drug that is abused more often than any other. Which drug?

▼ One drug kills more people than any other. Which one?

▼ Cigarettes can harm people who never smoke. How?

As you read this unit, think of ways to protect your health by saying no to drugs.

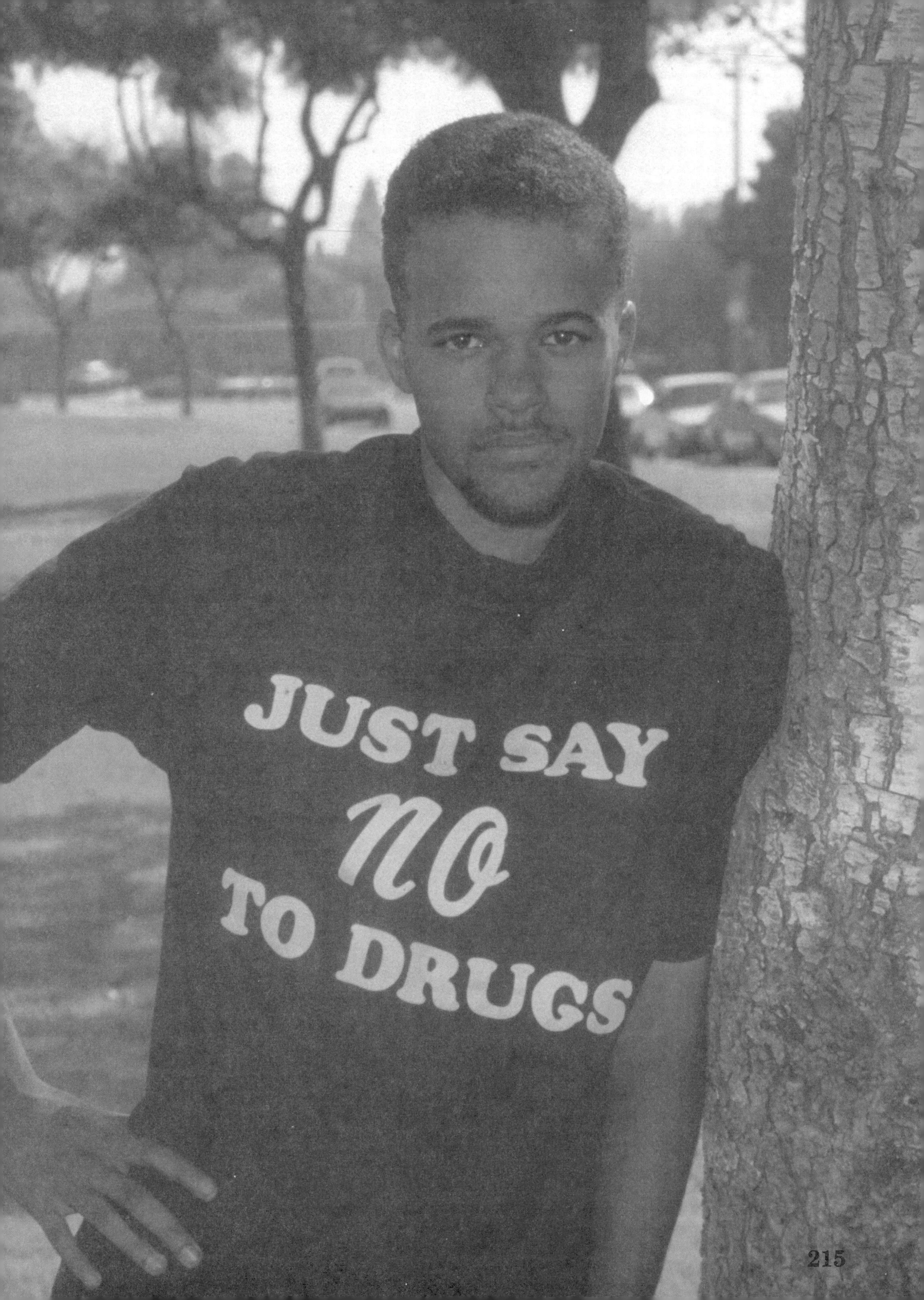
JUST SAY
NO
TO DRUGS

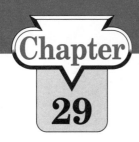

Chapter 29

Understanding Drug Abuse

Think About as You Read

- **What are the safe ways to take medicine?**
- **What are three types of drug abuse?**
- **Why do people abuse drugs?**

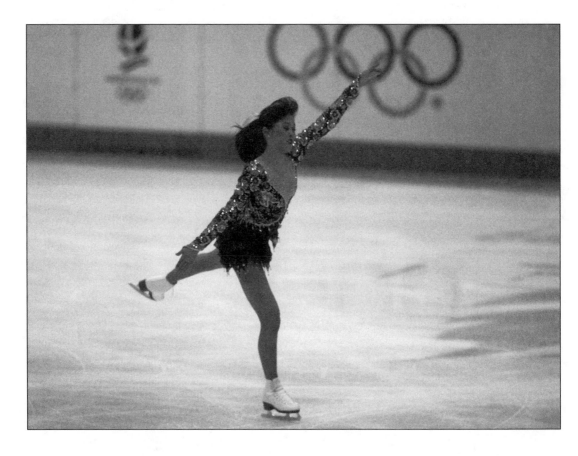

Kristi Yamaguchi never abused drugs. She wanted to reach her goal of winning a gold medal.

Skater Kristi Yamaguchi reached her goal in 1992. She won the gold medal for the United States at the Winter Olympics. Kristi had practiced many hours each day to become a skating star. One of the reasons she was able to reach her goal was that she never abused drugs. Kristi believes you must say no to drugs if you want to reach your goals.

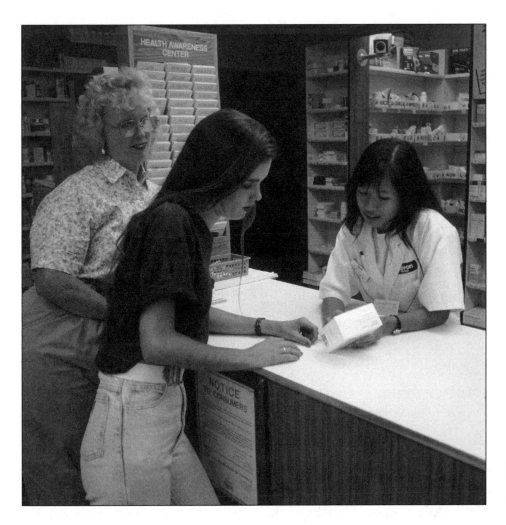

Some drugs are medicines that can be bought only with a prescription from a doctor.

What Are Drugs?

There are many kinds of drugs. A drug is a chemical or other substance that changes the way your body works. A drug can also affect your mind, feelings, and actions. Most drugs cure, try to cure, or prevent diseases.

Some drugs are medicines, such as antibiotics. You may need a prescription to buy some medicines. You can buy other medicines, such as aspirin, without a prescription.

There are also dangerous drugs. Many of these drugs are illegal. It is against the law to buy, sell, make, or use illegal drugs. **Heroin** is an illegal drug.

Heroin is a dangerous, habit-forming drug.

Using Medicine Safely

There are two groups of medicines. There are prescription drugs and over-the-counter drugs.

217

You can buy prescription drugs only with a prescription from a doctor. Antibiotics are one kind of prescription drug. Read and follow the directions on the label. Be sure to take the drug. Tell your doctor if you have **side effects** from taking the drug. Do not share your medicine with others. You should never take another person's prescription drug. The drug may be dangerous for you.

Always follow your doctor's directions when taking prescribed medicine. If you are sick, your doctor may tell you to take an antibiotic for ten days. You may not get well if you take it for less than ten days.

You do not need a prescription to buy an over-the-counter drug. If you are taking a prescription drug, check with your doctor before using an over-the-counter drug. Use over-the-counter drugs correctly. Read labels on over-the-counter drugs. Follow the directions. Pay attention to warnings and possible side effects. Do not use medicine after the **expiration date** on the label has passed. Never use medicine if the seal is broken when you buy it. Never drink alcohol when you take medicine.

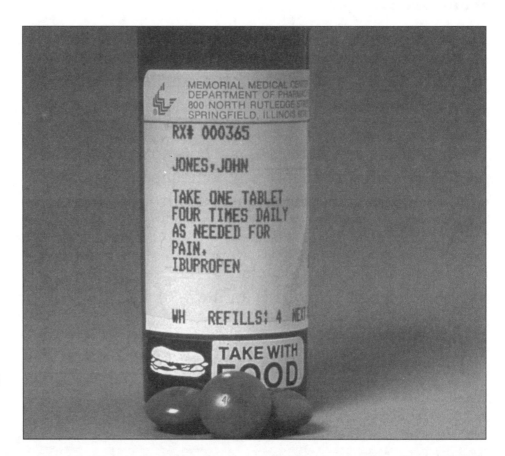

Your medicine has a label with directions. Always read and follow those directions.

218

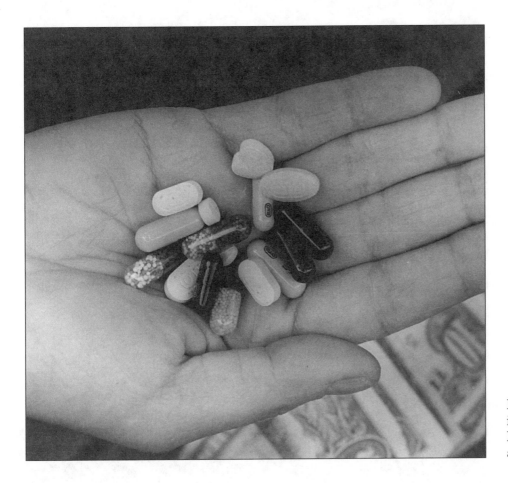

Drug abuse is using drugs in a way that is not correct. Many kinds of drugs are abused.

What Is Drug Abuse?

Drug abuse is using a drug in a way that is not correct. Drug abuse is also using a drug for no medical reason. There are three kinds of drug abuse. The first is when people do not take over-the-counter or prescription drugs correctly. Perhaps a person should take one pill three times a day. Instead the person takes all three pills at once. The second kind of drug abuse is the use of any illegal drug. The third type of drug abuse is when people take prescription drugs that belong to someone else.

How Does Abusing Drugs Harm People?

People who abuse drugs can develop a strong **dependence** on them. People with physical dependence must have drugs for their bodies to feel normal. People with emotional dependence must use drugs to avoid having certain unpleasant feelings. Dependence makes it very hard to stop using drugs.

Dependence is the very strong need for drugs.

219

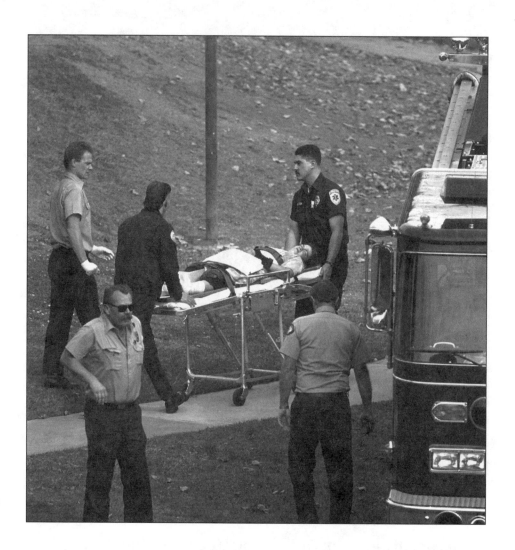

Some people take large amounts of a drug. This can be very dangerous.

Tolerance means the body needs more of a drug to get the same feeling it once felt with smaller amounts.

To feel **high** means to have a good feeling that lasts a short time. People sometimes get high from abusing drugs.

People who abuse drugs develop **tolerance**. People may feel **high** from taking a small amount of a drug. Later they need to take more of the drug to feel good. Taking large amounts of a drug can be dangerous. It can cause death.

Many people use needles to get drugs such as heroin into their bodies. They often share their needles with other drug abusers. Sharing needles can spread AIDS. Sharing needles can also spread other dangerous diseases that may cause death.

You break the law when you buy, sell, make, or use illegal drugs. You may go to jail.

Illegal drugs are very expensive. A drug abuser can spend hundreds of dollars a day to buy drugs. Most drug abusers do not have the money they need to buy their drugs. They may kill and steal to get money. Some drug abusers sell drugs to get money.

Why Do People Abuse Drugs?

Here are five reasons people abuse drugs.

1. People abuse drugs because of peer pressure. They decide to abuse drugs because others are doing it.
2. People abuse drugs to deal with stress. They abuse drugs to forget their problems.
3. People may abuse drugs because they want to know how the drug will make them feel.
4. Some people do not have friends. They think abusing drugs will help them make friends with other drug abusers.
5. People abuse drugs to show they do not have to listen to their parents or other people who make rules.

Who Abuses Drugs?

Most drug abusers are unhappy people without goals. They have low self-esteem. Their own friends may abuse drugs.

You can often tell when people are abusing drugs. Their behavior may suddenly change. Getting and abusing drugs is their main goal in life. They may no longer care about their family and friends. They may stop caring about their appearance.

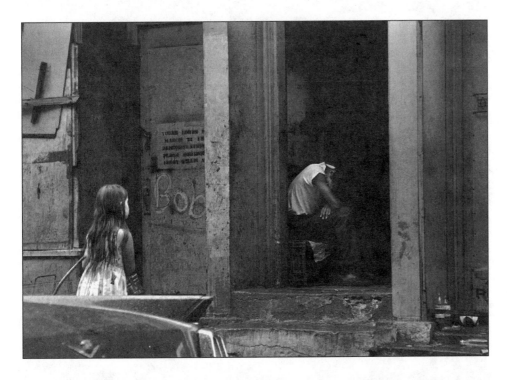

Drug abusers don't care about many things. Their main goal is to get and abuse drugs.

221

Drug abusers may stop caring about their schoolwork. They may skip classes. Their grades may be lower. Many drug abusers drop out of school.

Drug abusers say they can stop using drugs at any time. But a drug habit is hard to break. Drug abusers usually need help to get off and stay off drugs.

How to Feel Good Without Drugs

People with good emotional health do not need to abuse drugs to feel good. They do enjoyable activities to feel good. Listening to music or working on a hobby are ways to feel good. Other people like running, swimming, and riding a bike. Some people join clubs. Many people enjoy spending time with close friends who do not abuse drugs.

All people have stress in their lives. Using drugs is a dangerous way to handle stress. Exercising and getting enough rest are better ways. Talking about your problems with a trusted adult is a healthy way to handle stress.

Find ways to feel good without abusing drugs. Always remember that drugs can ruin your life.

People can feel good without using drugs. Exercising is one good way to handle stress.

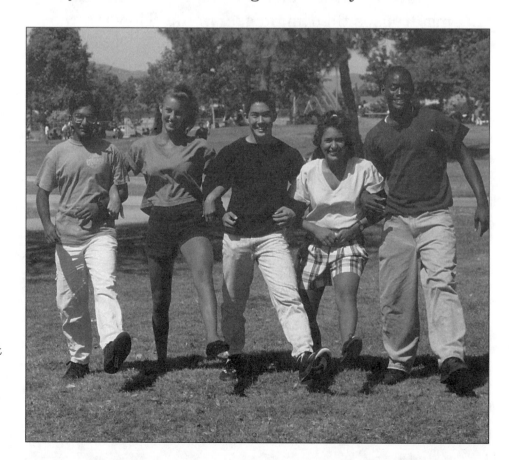

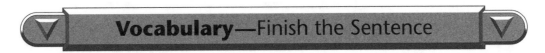

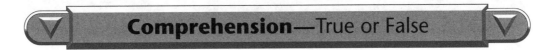

Vocabulary—Finish the Sentence

Choose a word or words from the box to complete each sentence. Write the correct answers on your paper.

drug abuse	high
dependence	side effects

1. Tell your doctor if you have any _____ from a prescription medicine.

2. Using a drug in a way that is not correct is _____ .

3. People who must have drugs to feel normal have a physical and emotional _____ on the drugs.

4. Sometimes people abuse drugs to feel _____ .

Comprehension—True or False

Write **True** on your paper for each sentence that is true. Write **False** on your paper for each sentence that is false. There are two false sentences. Rewrite the false sentences on your paper to make them true.

1. A drug is a chemical or other substance that changes the way your body works.

2. Illegal drugs do not cost very much.

3. Drug abusers who build up a tolerance need less of the drug to feel good.

4. You should read the labels on all medicines.

5. Sharing needles can lead to AIDS.

6. You break the law if you buy, sell, make, or use illegal drugs.

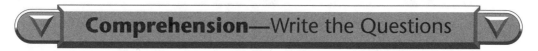

Using What You Learned

Comprehension—Write the Questions

Below are the answers for some questions from this chapter. Read each answer. Then write on your paper a possible question to go with each answer. Use the question words to help you.

1. Who _____ ?

   A doctor writes prescriptions for prescription drugs.

2. What _____ ?

   People who abuse drugs can develop a strong dependence on them.

3. What _____ ?

   Exercising and getting enough rest are good ways to handle stress.

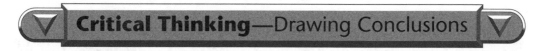

Critical Thinking—Drawing Conclusions

Read the paragraph. Then use the six steps below to decide what to do about drug abuse. Write complete sentences on your paper to answer each question.

Imagine that your best friend is thinking about trying some illegal drugs. Your friend wants you to try them, too. On your way home from a movie, your friend shows you the illegal drugs.

Step 1. What is the problem?

Step 2. What are two ways to solve the problem?

Step 3. What is one consequence for each choice listed in Step 2?

Step 4. Which choice do you think is best?

Step 5. What can you do to put your decision into action?

Step 6. Think about your decision. Why was this the best choice for you?

The Abuse of Drugs

Think About as You Read

• What are the dangers of marijuana, heroin, and cocaine?

• How can you say no to abusing drugs?

• Where can drug addicts get help?

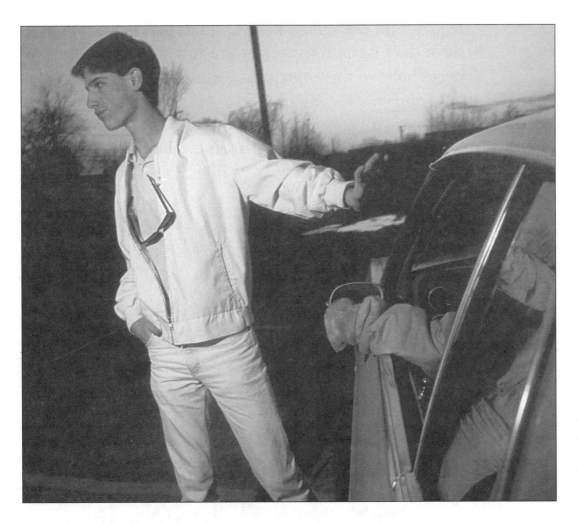

An important goal is to finish school. Reach your goals by always saying no to drugs.

Ramón's goal is to finish high school. It is not an easy goal. He knows he cannot reach his goal if he abuses drugs. Ramón always says no when someone asks him to abuse drugs.

Which Drugs Are Abused?

Codeine is a prescription drug that reduces pain.

Tranquilizers are prescription drugs that have a calming effect because they slow down the nervous system.

Doses are amounts of medicine that a person takes at one time.

Codeine and **tranquilizers** are prescription drugs. Some people abuse these drugs. They take much larger **doses** than their doctors order.

People use **marijuana** more than any other illegal drug. People often smoke it to feel high. But marijuana does not always give people a good feeling.

Marijuana can make people forget things. People who use marijuana may care less about reaching their goals. The drug makes people think and act more slowly. People who are using the drug find it hard to ride a bike or drive a car. Marijuana smoke can cause lung cancer.

Marijuana can cause emotional dependence. People believe they must use marijuana to feel good. Some experts believe that marijuana is often the first drug people abuse.

A **narcotic** is a drug that reduces pain and causes dependence.

Heroin is a very dangerous drug. It is a **narcotic**. You can buy a mild narcotic such as codeine with a prescription. Heroin is always illegal.

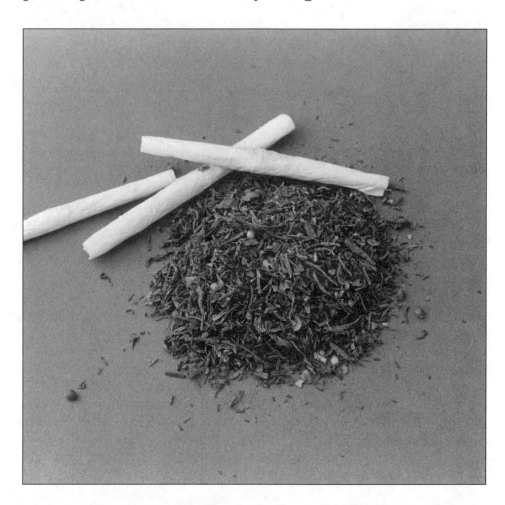

It is against the law to smoke marijuana. People think and act more slowly when taking the drug.

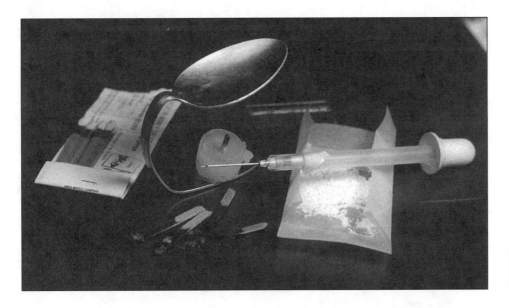

Some people inject heroin into their veins. Many of these people become addicts.

Heroin causes terrible dependence problems. At first heroin makes people feel happy and high. Then people develop emotional and physical dependence on it. They stop feeling high. But they must have the drug to feel normal. Heroin users become **addicts** because their need for heroin is so strong. Heroin addicts have only one goal. That goal is to have enough heroin to feel normal.

Heroin addicts develop tolerance for the drug. They need larger and larger doses of it. Sometimes very large doses kill an addict.

Heroin addicts go through **withdrawal** pains when they do not have the drug. They need medical help to stop using heroin.

Cocaine and **crack** are other illegal drugs. They are **stimulants**. At first they make people feel very happy. But the drugs later make people feel very sad. They use more cocaine and crack to feel happy again. Cocaine and crack abusers have dependence on these drugs. They must have them to feel happy. They develop tolerance for the drugs.

Withdrawal from cocaine and crack is hard. People feel tired and sad. They may become angry easily. They often get into fights. People who abuse cocaine and crack may have a strong need for the drugs for many months after they stop using them.

Addicts are people with such strong dependence on drugs that they cannot stop using them.

Withdrawal is the body's reaction to not having a drug.

Cocaine is an illegal drug that speeds up the nervous system. Its effects last a short time.

Crack is a strong form of cocaine. People smoke crack.

Stimulants are drugs that speed up the body's systems.

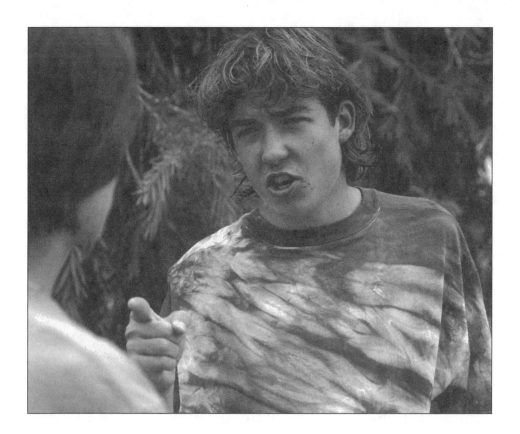

Hallucinogens can make people get angry easily.

The Abuse of Hallucinogens and Inhalants

Hallucinogens are drugs that make people see, hear, taste, and smell things differently. Colors and sounds seem different. LSD and PCP are hallucinogens. Angel dust is another name for PCP.

Hallucinogens make people see and hear things that are not real. These drugs can make things look scary and ugly. A string may look like a dangerous snake to a person who is using these drugs.

People feel less pain when they are using hallucinogens. They may burn or cut themselves and not know they are hurt.

Hallucinogens can make people feel very strong and powerful. So they take dangerous risks. Some drug abusers have jumped out of windows. Others become angry easily.

Hallucinogens are different from other drugs. They stay in the body's fat cells for many months. Since the drug stays in the body, it can start to work again many months later. People may see and hear things again that are not real. They may use risk behaviors again.

Hallucinogens can damage the brain. People using hallucinogens sometimes cannot think or speak clearly. They forget things. People develop emotional dependence on these drugs. They feel they must use them. Hallucinogens can cause death.

Inhalants are another group of drugs. You can buy many inhalants in stores. Spray paint, nail polish, airplane glue, and paint remover are inhalants. They become dangerous drugs when people abuse them in order to have pleasant feelings.

At first inhalants can make people feel relaxed and happy. People might feel dizzy later. They often throw up. They can have nosebleeds. People develop emotional dependence on inhalants. They must keep using them to feel good.

People develop tolerance for inhalants. So people must breathe in larger amounts to feel relaxed. Inhalants harm the body. They damage the lungs and the brain. They make the heart beat more slowly. People breathe much more slowly after abusing these drugs. People can die if inhalants make them stop breathing.

Look at the charts on pages 290–293. These charts list other drugs that people often abuse.

People sniff **inhalants** in order to have pleasant feelings.

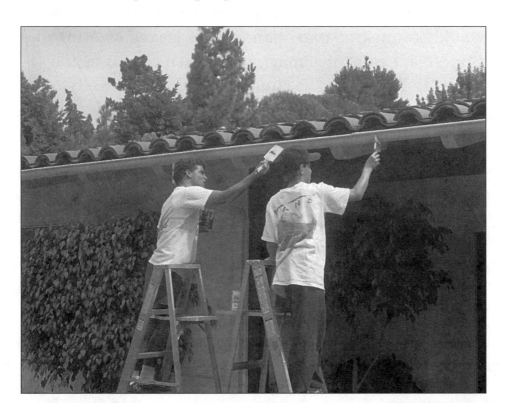

Some people abuse paint by inhaling it. Inhalants can make you feel dizzy.

229

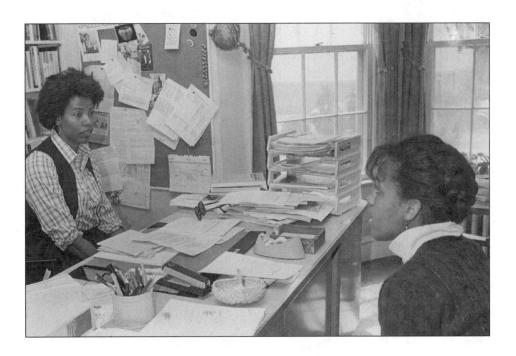

If someone asks you to abuse drugs, you can talk to a trusted adult about it.

Saying No to Drugs

Use these refusal skills to say no if someone asks you to abuse drugs.

1. Look at the person and say no. Tell why.
2. Suggest another activity in place of abusing drugs.
3. Walk away if the person pressures you.
4. Tell a parent or trusted adult.

Kelly used refusal skills. Anne invited Kelly to go to a party. Anne and Kelly knew the people at the party would be smoking marijuana. Kelly looked at Anne and said, "No, I won't use marijuana. Let's go to a movie instead." Anne tried to change Kelly's mind. Kelly walked away from Anne. Later that night Kelly talked to her father about what happened.

People who abuse drugs may ask you again and again to try drugs. Drug abusers may tell you that everyone uses drugs. They may say you are not part of the group if you do not use drugs.

Protect yourself from peer pressure to abuse drugs. Remember these four rules.

1. Do not abuse drugs even once. Abusing drugs can ruin your life.
2. Choose friends who do not abuse drugs.

3. Know that real friends do not want you to harm yourself with drugs.

4. Stay away from places where people abuse drugs.

Help for Drug Abusers

It is very hard for most drug abusers to stop abusing drugs. They must really want to stop.

To change their habits, drug abusers must stop using all drugs. When they stop using the drugs, abusers may have withdrawal pains. People often need medical care when they stop abusing drugs. Abusers can get help at drug treatment centers and special clinics. People can get information on how to stop abusing drugs from a school nurse or their doctor. They can also call a drug hot line.

Drug abusers should learn new ways to solve problems. They must learn decision-making skills. They need refusal skills to help them say no to drugs.

Feel good about yourself without abusing drugs. By saying no to drugs, you can have a healthier life.

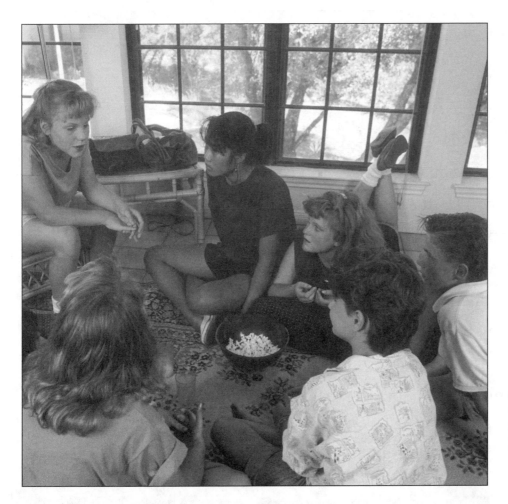

At drug treatment centers, drug abusers learn how to make decisions and solve problems.

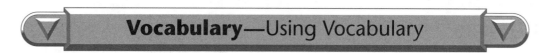

Using What You Learned

Vocabulary—Using Vocabulary

Use each word to write a complete sentence on your paper about drug abuse.

1. narcotic
2. stimulant
3. withdrawal
4. addicts
5. doses

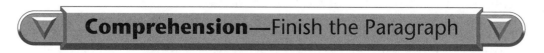

Comprehension—Finish the Paragraph

Number your paper from 1 to 9. Use a word from the box to finish each sentence. Write the correct answers on your paper.

prescription	pressure	abuse
cocaine	withdrawal	dependence
refusal	no	clinics

Sometimes people you know will try to get you to __(1)__ drugs. They may use peer __(2)__ to talk you into abusing drugs. You can use __(3)__ skills to protect yourself. Be sure to say __(4)__ if someone asks you to abuse drugs. Stay away from places where people abuse drugs.

Tranquilizers are drugs that can be bought with a __(5)__ . Other drugs, such as __(6)__ , are illegal. Some people have such a strong physical and emotional __(7)__ on drugs that they become addicts. Addicts develop tolerance for drugs.

When drug abusers stop using drugs, they may have __(8)__ pains. Addicts might need medical help to stop abusing drugs. Abusers can get help at drug treatment centers and special __(9)__ .

232

Comprehension—Write the Answer

Write a sentence on your paper to answer each question.

1. What illegal drug is used more than any other illegal drug?

2. How do people abuse prescription drugs?

3. Why do heroin users become addicts?

4. What kind of drugs are cocaine and crack?

5. What can hallucinogens damage?

6. Where can drug abusers get help?

Critical Thinking—Categories

Read the words in each group. Decide how they are alike. Find the best title in the box for each group. Write the title on your paper.

Inhalants	Drug Addict	Marijuana
Refusal Skills	Heroin	Hallucinogens

1. causes lung cancer
   makes people forgetful
   slows thinking and movement

2. dependence problems
   narcotic
   illegal drug

3. PCP and LSD
   cause brain damage
   people see and hear things that
      are not real

4. can cause nosebleeds
   harm the lungs and brain
   spray paint, nail polish, airplane glue

5. dependent on a drug
   has poor decision-making skills
   may die from large doses of a drug

6. say no
   stay away from people who abuse drugs
   don't go to places where drugs are
      abused

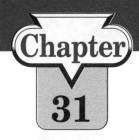

Alcohol and Health

Think About as You Read

- Why is alcohol a dangerous drug?
- Why do people drink alcohol?
- How can alcoholics be helped?

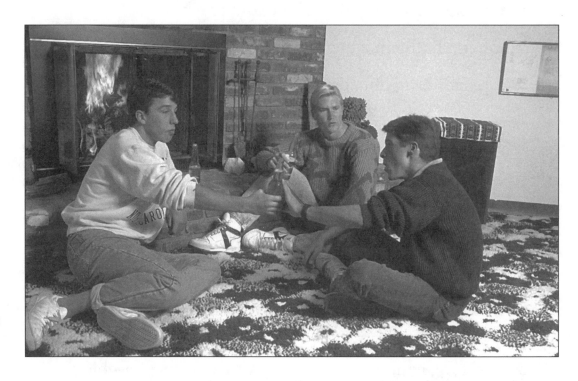

Alcohol is a dangerous drug. You can say no when people ask you to drink alcohol.

Jason went to a party. Many people were drinking beer. His friends tried to get him to drink some beer. Jason used refusal skills to say no to his friends. Later he left the party. Jason had decided that he would not drink alcohol.

Alcohol Is a Dangerous Drug

More people use alcohol than any other drug. Alcohol comes in many types of drinks. Beer, wine, and liquor have alcohol in them.

Every state has made alcohol illegal for people under a certain age. In the United States, you must be at least 21 years old to buy and use alcohol. Teen-agers who buy alcohol are breaking the law.

When a person drinks alcohol, it quickly goes into the blood. The blood carries alcohol to every cell in the body. Alcohol is a **depressant**. It changes the way the brain works.

A **depressant** is a drug that slows down the nervous system.

Alcohol slows down the messages that the brain sends through the nerves. Alcohol will slow down your thinking. You will not be able to think as clearly. Alcohol will slow down the way your body moves. This can cause you to have accidents. Drunk drivers cause more than half of all car accidents.

There are three main reasons why people abuse alcohol. Some people abuse it because they have low self-esteem. Other people are bored. They think it will be fun to get high on alcohol. Others want their friends who drink alcohol to accept them.

Drunk drivers cause more than half of all car accidents. Don't drink and drive.

Why Is Alcohol Harmful?

Abusing alcohol for a long period of time can harm your physical health. It can damage your brain, your heart, and your digestive system. It can destroy your liver and cause death.

Alcohol abuse harms your social health. People who abuse alcohol cannot work well with others in school or at their jobs. Some people who abuse alcohol get into fights.

Alcohol abuse harms your emotional health. Many people cannot control their feelings when they abuse alcohol. Alcohol stops them from making wise decisions. They are more likely to abuse other family members and friends, too.

Alcohol abuse causes physical and emotional dependence. People can develop tolerance for alcohol. They need to drink larger amounts to feel normal. Withdrawal is very painful.

If a pregnant female drinks, the alcohol can harm the unborn baby. Even small amounts of alcohol can harm the baby. But large amounts can damage the brain, the heart, and the body of an unborn baby.

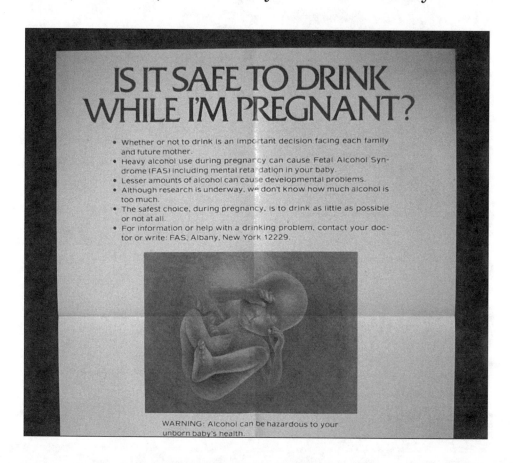

IS IT SAFE TO DRINK WHILE I'M PREGNANT?

- Whether or not to drink is an important decision facing each family and future mother.
- Heavy alcohol use during pregnancy can cause Fetal Alcohol Syndrome (FAS) including mental retardation in your baby.
- Lesser amounts of alcohol can cause developmental problems.
- Although research is underway, we don't know how much alcohol is too much.
- The safest choice, during pregnancy, is to drink as little as possible or not at all.
- For information or help with a drinking problem, contact your doctor or write: FAS, Albany, New York 12229.

WARNING: Alcohol can be hazardous to your unborn baby's health.

Alcohol can damage the brain, the heart, and the body of an unborn baby.

236

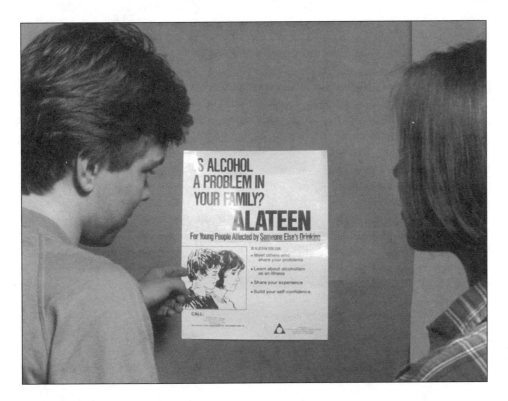

Alateen groups help teen-agers live with family members who are alcoholics.

Understanding and Treating Alcoholism

There are many people who cannot make wise decisions about using alcohol. They abuse alcohol even when it causes problems in their lives. Some cannot stop drinking once they start. These people suffer from the disease of **alcoholism**. They are **alcoholics**. About four million teen-agers have drinking problems.

Here are some signs of alcoholism.

1. The person is often drunk.
2. The person drinks alcohol in the morning.
3. The person does poor work at school or at work.
4. The person drinks secretly.
5. The person forgets many things.
6. The person needs larger amounts of alcohol.

There is no cure for alcoholism. Alcoholics control their disease by not drinking alcohol.

Many alcoholics need help to stop drinking. They need to get help from a doctor or treatment program. Doctors and treatment programs can help alcoholics withdraw from alcohol. Alcoholics also need to learn better ways to solve problems. They need to learn to make wise decisions and use refusal skills.

Alcoholism is a disease in which a person's need to drink alcohol is strong. The person cannot control the need to drink.

237

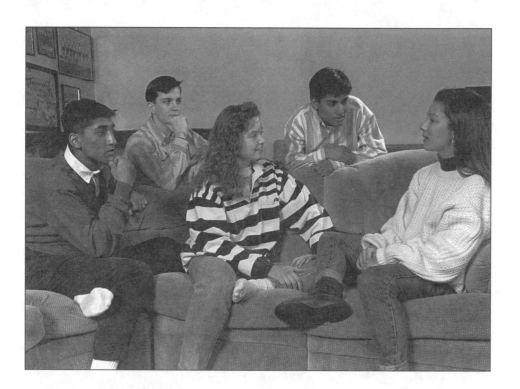

Teens make wise decisions when they choose friends who do not drink alcohol.

Recovering alcoholics have learned how to stop drinking alcohol.

Alcoholics Anonymous is a group of recovering alcoholics who help each other avoid alcohol.

Recovering alcoholics must never drink alcohol again. They need help from groups like **Alcoholics Anonymous**. Members help each other avoid alcohol. Other groups help teen-agers stop drinking.

Saying No to Alcohol

Alcohol will not be a problem for you if you never use it. It takes only one drink for many people to become alcoholics.

Many teen-agers drink alcohol because their friends do. Teens are making wise decisions when they choose friends who do not drink alcohol.

Anita used refusal skills when her friend Julie asked her to drink beer. Anita said, "No, Julie, I don't drink alcohol. Let's have a soda instead." Julie laughed at Anita and made fun of her decision. Then Julie tried to change Anita's mind. Anita left. She later talked to her mother about what had happened. Anita and her mother felt Anita had made a good decision.

Some decisions are harder to make than others. You are making a wise decision if you never use alcohol. Your decision will help you have good health and wellness.

238

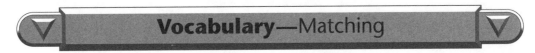

Vocabulary—Matching

Match each vocabulary word in **Group B** with a sentence from **Group A** that tells about the word. Write the letter of the correct answer on your paper.

Group A

1. This disease cannot be cured, but it can be controlled if the person stops drinking alcohol.

2. These people often need help from a doctor or treatment center to stop drinking alcohol.

3. This drug slows down the nervous system.

4. These people used to drink, but they have learned to say no to alcohol.

5. The members of this group help one another avoid drinking alcohol.

Group B

a. alcoholics

b. Alcoholics Anonymous

c. alcoholism

d. recovering alcoholics

e. alcohol

Comprehension—True or False

Write **True** on your paper for each sentence that is true. Write **False** on your paper for each sentence that is false. There are two false sentences. Rewrite the false sentences on your paper to make them true.

1. More people use alcohol than any other drug.

2. Some states have not made alcohol illegal for people under a certain age.

3. Alcohol can slow down the way the body moves.

4. Alcohol cannot harm your physical, social, and emotional health.

5. Alcoholics Anonymous is a group that helps recovering alcoholics.

239

Comprehension—Writing About Health

Answer the following question in complete sentences on your paper.

What are five signs of alcoholism?

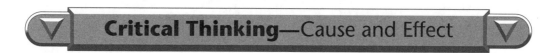

Critical Thinking—Cause and Effect

Write sentences on your paper by matching each cause on the left with an effect on the right.

Cause

1. You use refusal skills to say no to beer, wine, and liquor, so _____

2. Alcohol slows down the way the body moves, so _____

3. Many alcoholics cannot stop drinking without help, so _____

4. There is no cure for alcoholism, so _____

5. The blood carries alcohol, so _____

6. Steve has a physical and emotional dependence on alcohol, so _____

7. Stacy drank large amounts of alcohol during her pregnancy, so _____

Effect

a. alcohol can cause people to have accidents.

b. he drinks larger amounts of alcohol just to feel normal.

c. many alcoholics get help from a doctor or treatment program.

d. you avoid developing a drinking problem.

e. alcoholics must control their disease by not drinking.

f. her baby has many health problems.

g. alcohol quickly goes to every cell in the body.

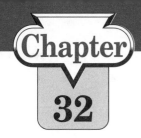

Tobacco and Health

| Think About as You Read |

- **Why is tobacco harmful?**
- **How does cigarette smoke hurt people who do not smoke?**
- **Why do people smoke?**

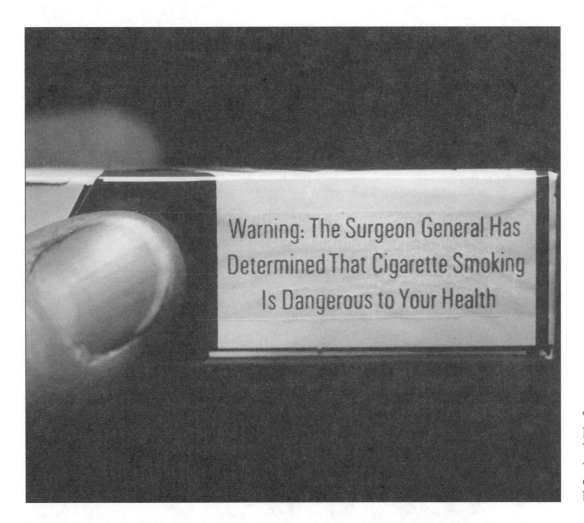

Tobacco is a harmful drug. You can find a warning label on every cigarette box.

Would you spend $400 or more a year on something that could make you very sick? Millions of people do. They spend money to buy cigarettes. They harm their health with tobacco.

241

How Does Tobacco Hurt People?

More people die each year of health problems caused by the use of tobacco than from any other drug. Most tobacco is smoked in cigarettes. Some people chew, dip, or sniff **smokeless tobacco**. All types of tobacco can harm your health.

There are many dangerous chemicals in tobacco. The most dangerous is **nicotine**. Nicotine is a poison. It is also a stimulant. It makes the heart beat faster. It raises blood pressure. People who use tobacco have more heart attacks and heart diseases than people who do not use tobacco.

Nicotine causes dependence. Smokers need it to feel good. Nicotine makes it hard to stop smoking.

Tobacco can harm the unborn babies of pregnant females who smoke. Nicotine travels through the umbilical cord to the baby. It can cause the unborn baby to be born too early. Pregnant females who smoke often have smaller babies that are less healthy.

Smokeless tobacco is made from tobacco leaves and is chewed, dipped, or sniffed.

Nicotine is a drug in tobacco that causes dependence.

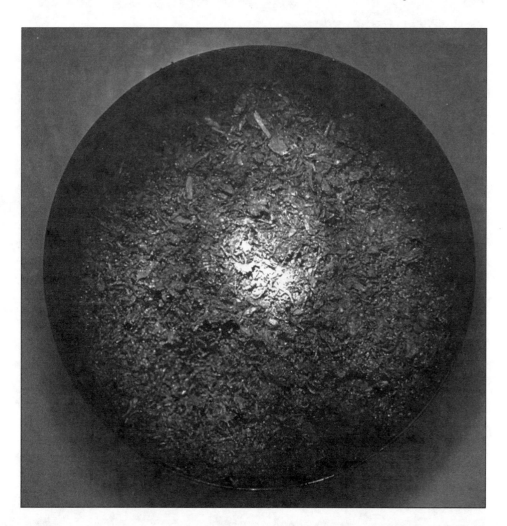

People chew, dip, or sniff smokeless tobacco. All tobacco is harmful to your health.

242

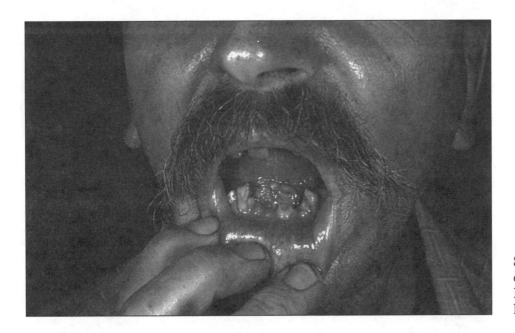

Smoking cigarettes can cause cancer in the mouth. It causes lip, throat, and lung cancer.

Tobacco is harmful in seven other ways.

1. Smokers may have very bad coughs.
2. Smokers become short of breath and feel tired more easily than people who do not smoke.
3. Smokers have more heart and lung diseases than people who do not smoke.
4. Smokers are more likely to get lung cancer.
5. Smokers get more mouth, lip, and throat cancers. They get other cancers more often.
6. Tobacco harms the teeth. It also makes ugly, yellow stains on teeth.
7. Smokers cause more fires in their homes.

Smoking Harms People Who Do Not Smoke

Cigarettes can harm you even if you never smoke. When people smoke cigarettes, tobacco smoke goes into the air. The smoke in the air is **sidestream smoke**. If you are in a room with people who are smoking, you are breathing sidestream smoke. You are a **passive smoker** when you breathe tobacco smoke.

Sidestream smoke is full of dangerous chemicals. People who live or work with smokers have to breathe these dangerous chemicals. Passive smokers develop lung disease and lung cancer more often than people who breathe clean air.

Sidestream smoke is the smoke sent into the air by the burning end of a cigarette, pipe, or cigar.

A **passive smoker** breathes smoke from cigarettes, pipes, or cigars.

243

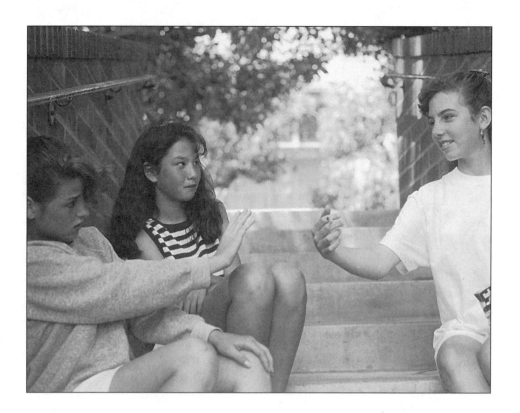

Use refusal skills to say no to smoking. You can say, "No. I don't smoke."

Many public places protect people from sidestream smoke. Most offices and restaurants have separate areas for smokers. Many places no longer allow smoking.

Why Do People Use Tobacco?

Each year many people start to smoke. Most of these new smokers are teen-agers.

People may smoke for five different reasons. First, some people smoke because they are copying the behavior of family members who smoke. Second, they think smoking cigarettes will help them deal with stress. Third, some people smoke because of peer pressure. They want to fit in with their friends. Fourth, they want to show that they do not have to listen to others who are against smoking.

The fifth reason many people smoke is that they have low self-esteem. Some cigarette ads suggest smoking cigarettes makes you popular or good-looking. People with low self-esteem want to be like the people in the ads. Smoking makes them feel more important, grown up, or better looking.

Saying No to Tobacco

You know about the dangers of smoking. Here are three reasons to say no to tobacco.

1. It is illegal in the United States to smoke if you are under the age of 18.
2. You want to protect your health.
3. You do not want to waste your money on tobacco.

Saying no to smoking will raise your self-esteem. You will feel good about making a healthy decision. Choose friends who do not use tobacco. They will not ask you to smoke.

Use refusal skills to say no to smoking. The chart on this page shows five ways you can say no to smoking.

People who smoke can stop smoking. The body does get used to not having nicotine. The heart and lungs of a person who quits smoking can become healthier. People who want to stop smoking can ask for help from their doctor or school nurse.

The best way to take care of your health is by saying no to tobacco. You can reach your goal of wellness by not starting to use tobacco.

Saying No to Smoking

A Smoker May Say:	You Can Say:
1. Try a cigarette. These are great.	1. No. I don't use tobacco. OR—No. I don't smoke.
2. Everyone smokes.	2. No. I don't smoke because it is dangerous to my health.
3. Let's go to my house. We can smoke there.	3. No. I don't smoke. Let's go to a movie instead.
4. I don't want to be your friend if you don't smoke.	4. I don't need friends who smoke. I have good friends who don't smoke.
5. I really wish you would try my cigarettes.	5. If you were really my friend, you would not ask me to do something to harm my health.

Using What You Learned

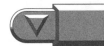

Vocabulary—Find the Meaning

Write on your paper the word or words that best complete each sentence.

1. When you breathe another person's tobacco smoke, you are a _____ .
   dangerous chemical   **passive smoker**   **member**

2. The dangerous stimulant found in tobacco is _____ .
   nicotine   **cancer**   **smoke**

3. If you are in a smoke-filled room, you are breathing _____ .
   lung cancer   **smokeless tobacco**   **sidestream smoke**

4. All types of tobacco, including _____ , can cause health problems.
   smokeless tobacco   **lung disease**   **blood pressure**

5. Cigarette _____ try to make people think that smoking will make them more popular or better looking.
   chemicals   **ads**   **fires**

Comprehension—Write the Questions

Below are the answers for some questions from this chapter. Read each answer. Then write on your paper a possible question to go with each answer. Use the question words to help you.

1. Why _____ ?

   Smoking is dangerous to the unborn baby of a pregnant female because it can cause the baby to be born too early and to be less healthy.

2. How _____ ?

   Many public places protect people from sidestream smoke by having separate areas for smokers or by not allowing smoking.

246

3. Why _____ ?

   It is dangerous to be around people who are smoking because the air will be filled with harmful chemicals.

4. What _____ ?

   The most dangerous chemical in tobacco is nicotine.

5. Who _____

   A doctor or school nurse can help you stop smoking.

6. How _____ ?

   You can reach your goal of wellness by not starting to use tobacco.

Critical Thinking—Fact or Opinion

Write **Fact** on your paper for each fact below. Write **Opinion** for each opinion. You should find four sentences that are opinions.

1. More people die each year from tobacco use than from any other drug.
2. All types of tobacco can harm your health.
3. Smoking should be illegal.
4. Smokers have more heart and lung diseases than people who do not smoke.
5. It is easy to quit smoking.
6. Smoking should not be allowed in any public place.
7. Tobacco can harm the unborn babies of pregnant females who smoke.
8. Passive smokers develop lung disease and lung cancer more often than people who breathe clean air.
9. Smoking is a good way to deal with stress.
10. Some people smoke because of peer pressure.

UNIT 10

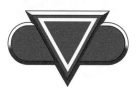

Fighting Disease

Modern medicine is helping people live longer, healthier lives. There are medicines that cure many diseases. Other medicines can prevent certain diseases. Doctors today have better tests and tools than in years past for learning what happens inside the body.

While doctors work at finding more cures for diseases, many people are using good health habits to stay well. Washing your hands often, exercising, and eating a healthy diet are a few things you can do to protect yourself from disease.

Have You Ever Wondered?

▼ Some diseases spread quickly from one person to another. How?
▼ A cold is very dangerous for a person with AIDS. Why?
▼ High blood pressure can cause other kinds of heart disease. Which ones?

As you read this unit, think about your own health habits. Learn what you can do to avoid disease and reach the goal of wellness.

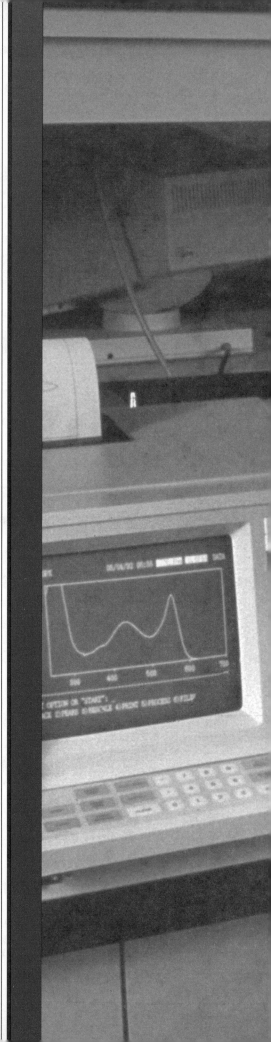

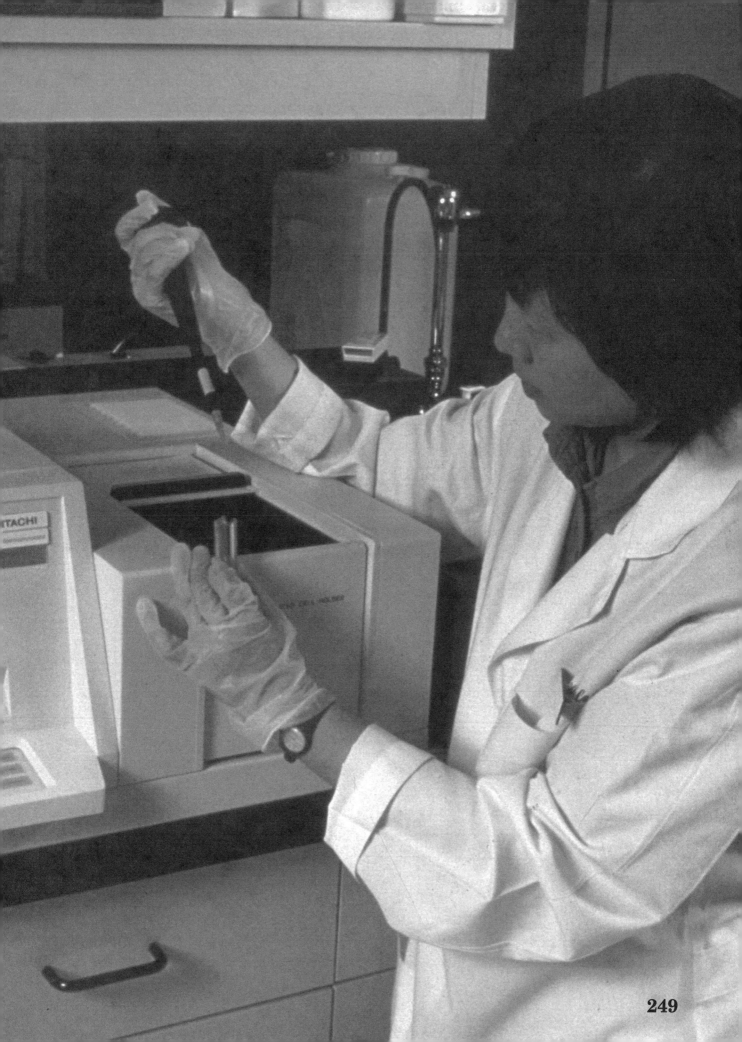

Chapter 33

Communicable Diseases

Think About as You Read

- How are communicable diseases spread among people?
- How does the body fight disease?
- How can you avoid disease?

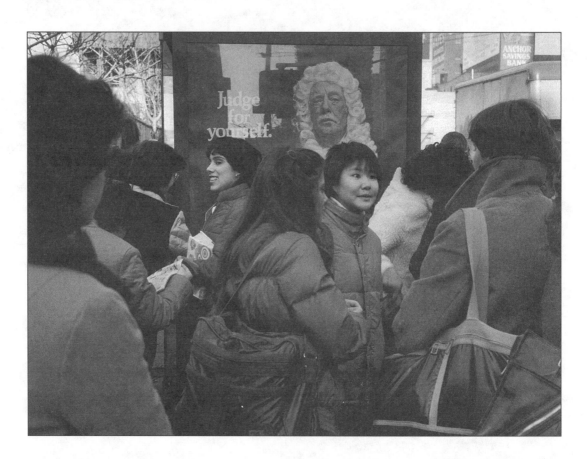

The flu is a communicable disease that spreads quickly during the winter.

A **virus** is a very tiny living thing that can cause diseases. A virus can multiply and grow only when it is inside the body's cells.

Every winter a few students in your school may get sick with the flu. Before long the flu may spread to other people in school. A **virus** causes this disease. The flu is one of the many **communicable diseases**. Communicable diseases spread from one person to another. In this chapter you will learn about the causes and treatments of these diseases.

The Cause and Spread of Communicable Diseases

Pathogens cause all communicable diseases. Bacteria and viruses are two types of pathogens.

Bacteria **reproduce** quickly inside your body. Antibiotics kill bacteria. As viruses reproduce, they destroy cells. Antibiotics do not kill most viruses.

Communicable diseases are spread in many ways.

1. Touching, hugging, or kissing a sick person can make you sick.
2. Using a sick person's face towel, dish, cup, or other object can make you sick.
3. When a sick person coughs or sneezes, small drops filled with pathogens go into the air. You can get sick from breathing these small drops.
4. You can get sick from eating food that is not cooked or stored in the right way.
5. There are pathogens inside some animals and insects. When animals or insects bite you, those pathogens enter your blood and can cause disease.
6. Flies and other insects often carry pathogens on their bodies. You can get sick from eating food or using dishes and objects that flies have touched.

Pathogens are very tiny living things that cause disease. They are too small to be seen without a microscope.

To **reproduce** means to make other living things. People reproduce by having babies. Bacteria make more bacteria when they reproduce.

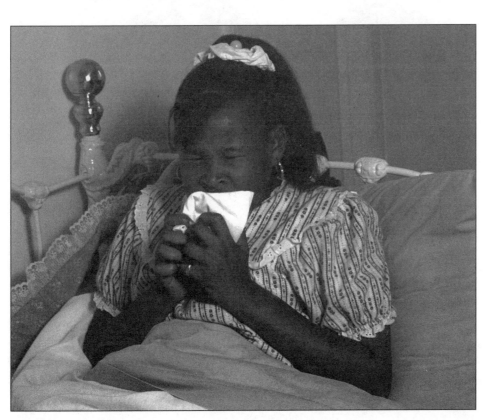

Using a sick person's towels, sheets, and cups can make you sick.

251

How the Body Fights Disease

Your body has three ways to fight disease. First, unbroken skin keeps most pathogens out of your body. Second, chemicals in your tears, mouth, and stomach kill pathogens. Third, your **immune system** fights disease. Different kinds of white blood cells make up your immune system. One kind of white blood cell makes **antibodies**. Antibodies kill pathogens. Your body makes different antibodies for different diseases.

Vaccines give your body **immunity** to certain diseases. Most vaccines give you immunity that lasts for as long as you live. Other vaccines do not give you lasting immunity. You must take these vaccines again after a number of years have passed. You get most vaccines in shots. You can swallow the polio vaccine.

Common Communicable Diseases

Many different viruses cause colds. Medicines do not cure colds. The best way to prevent colds is by washing your hands often with soap and warm water.

Vaccines are medicines that help the body make antibodies. Vaccines protect you from getting certain diseases.

Immunity means the body can fight off a disease without becoming sick.

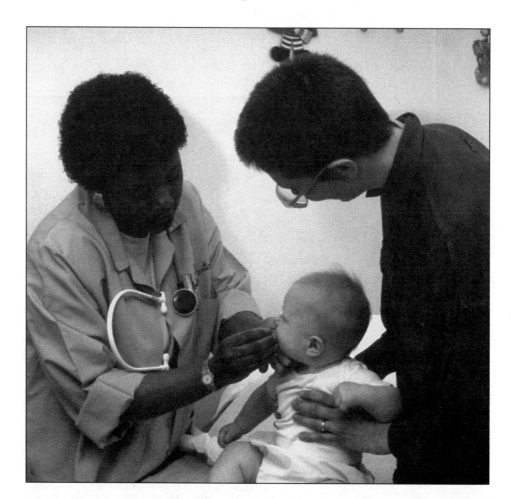

This baby is being given the polio vaccine. This vaccine can be swallowed.

Viruses or bacteria can cause sore throats. **Strep bacteria** cause many sore throats. A doctor will use a **throat culture** to learn which type of sore throat you have. The doctor will give you antibiotics to treat strep throat. Strep throat can cause heart and kidney damage if it is not treated. Always see a doctor if your sore throat lasts more than two days. See a doctor if you have a fever of 101° or higher.

The chart on page 254 provides information about other diseases.

A **throat culture** is the growth of bacteria from the throat. The bacteria grow in a small, closed dish.

Preventing Disease with Good Health Habits

You can protect yourself against communicable diseases. The most important way is by having all the vaccines you need.

Here are eight more health rules that can help you stay well.

1. Wash your hands with soap and warm water before you eat or cook. Wash them after you use the bathroom or change a baby's diaper.
2. Wash cuts with soap and warm water to keep germs out of your body.
3. After preparing raw meat or chicken, wash your hands, knives, and cooking tools with soap and warm water.
4. Use soap and warm water to wash all towels, dishes, and objects after a sick person uses them.
5. Try not to touch and kiss people who have communicable diseases.
6. Cover your nose and mouth with a tissue when you cough or sneeze. Then throw away that used tissue.
7. See a doctor to prevent small health problems from becoming big ones.
8. Take care of your health. Eat healthy foods. Exercise and get enough sleep.

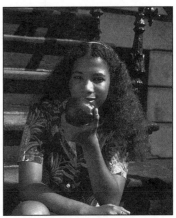

Eating healthy foods helps you protect yourself from communicable diseases.

Good health habits and vaccines can help you avoid communicable diseases. Good health habits and vaccines will help you reach your goal of wellness.

COMMON COMMUNICABLE DISEASES

Disease	Cause	Common Symptoms	Treatment
strep throat	strep bacteria	possible sore throat, fever, swollen glands in the neck	Take antibiotics, drink liquids, and take medicine for pain and body aches.
common cold	more than 100 different viruses	possible sore throat, runny nose, red eyes, cough	Get plenty of bed rest, eat a healthy diet, drink liquids, and take medicine for pain and body aches.
pneumonia	bacteria or viruses	infection and pain in lungs, chest pain, cough, difficulty breathing	Take antibiotics to treat pneumonia caused by bacteria. Get plenty of bed rest, drink fluids, and take medicine for pain and body aches.
flu	viruses	fever, muscle pain, headache, stomachache, sore throat	Get plenty of bed rest, eat a healthy diet, drink fluids, and take medicine for pain and body aches.
hepatitis A	viruses from unclean food or water	liver infection, fever, skin looks yellow, nausea (a sick feeling in the stomach), vomiting (throwing up)	Get plenty of bed rest and eat a healthy diet.
hepatitis B	viruses from infected blood and body fluids	liver infection, fever, skin looks yellow, nausea (a sick feeling in the stomach), vomiting (throwing up)	Get plenty of bed rest and eat a healthy diet.
tuberculosis	bacteria	coughing, coughing up blood, weight loss, feeling very tired, night sweats	Take antibiotics, eat a healthy diet, and get plenty of bed rest.
mononucleosis	viruses	sore throat, swollen glands in the neck, pain in joints, fever, feeling very tired	Eat a healthy diet, get plenty of bed rest, and take medicine for body aches.
chicken pox	viruses	rash, fever, aching muscles	Get plenty of bed rest, drink fluids, take baths, and take medicine for fever and itching.

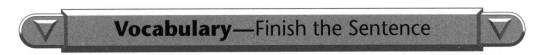

Using What You Learned

Choose a word or words from the box to complete each sentence. Write the correct answers on your paper.

reproduce	virus	immune system
pathogens	vaccines	antibodies

1. A _____ causes the flu.

2. Viruses and bacteria are types of _____ that can cause communicable diseases.

3. White blood cells make _____ to kill pathogens.

4. Viruses destroy cells as they _____ .

5. White blood cells are part of your _____ .

6. You get most _____ in shots.

Comprehension—Write the Questions

Below are the answers for some questions from this chapter. Read each answer. Then write on your paper a possible question to go with each answer. Use the question words to help you.

1. Where _____ ?

   Bacteria reproduce in the body.

2. How _____ ?

   Communicable diseases can be spread by touching a sick person.

3. How _____ ?

   Unbroken skin helps your body fight disease by keeping pathogens out of your body.

255

4. Why _____ ?

You should get a throat culture to find out what type of sore throat you have.

5. How _____ ?

You can prevent many communicable diseases by having all of the vaccines you need.

6. What _____ ?

Cover your nose and mouth with a tissue when you cough or sneeze.

7. What _____ ?

Your immune system fights disease.

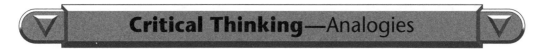

Critical Thinking—Analogies

Use a word or words in the box to finish each sentence. Write the correct answers on your paper.

infected blood	**antibodies**	**pathogens**
strep bacteria	**tuberculosis**	**virus**

1. Virus is to flu as _____ are to some sore throats.

2. Cold is to communicable disease as _____ is to pathogen.

3. Vaccines are to immunity as _____ are to communicable diseases.

4. The immune system is to fighting disease as _____ are to killing pathogens.

5. Unclean food is to hepatitis A as _____ is to hepatitis B.

6. Mononucleosis is to sore throat as _____ is to coughing.

AIDS and STDs

Think About as You Read

- How do people get AIDS?
- How can people protect themselves from STDs and AIDS?
- How does AIDS harm the body?

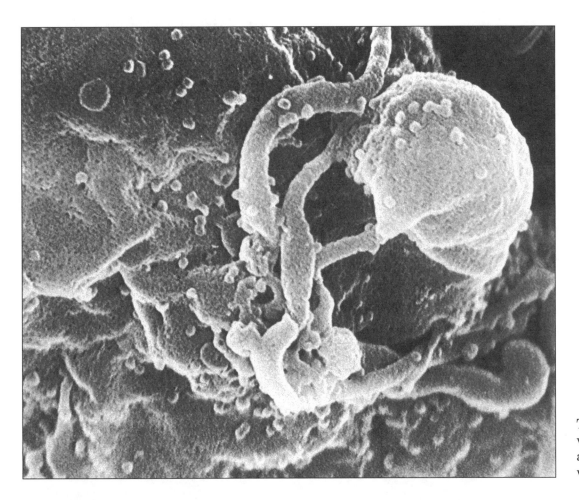

This is the AIDS virus. It attacks and destroys white blood cells.

Magic Johnson is a famous basketball star who has the AIDS virus. Magic Johnson now tells people to protect themselves from AIDS. In this chapter you will learn about AIDS and other sexually transmitted diseases, or STDs.

What Are Sexually Transmitted Diseases?

STDs are communicable diseases. To prevent STDs, avoid intimate sexual behavior.

Some STDs can be treated and cured with antibiotics and other medicines. If STDs are not treated, they can damage your body. You can die from STDs. A pregnant female can pass STDs to her unborn baby.

Chlamydia is the most common STD. One of its **symptoms** is **discharge** from the sex organs. Pregnant females who have chlamydia can pass the disease to their unborn babies. A baby born to a mother with chlamydia may have **pneumonia** and eye infections.

Learn about four STDs from the chart on page 259. Many people do not have symptoms until their bodies are badly damaged. Infected people can spread their disease to others.

Chlamydia is an STD that is caused by bacteria.

Symptoms are signs of a disease.

Discharge comes out of an infected part of the body.

Pneumonia is an infection of the lungs.

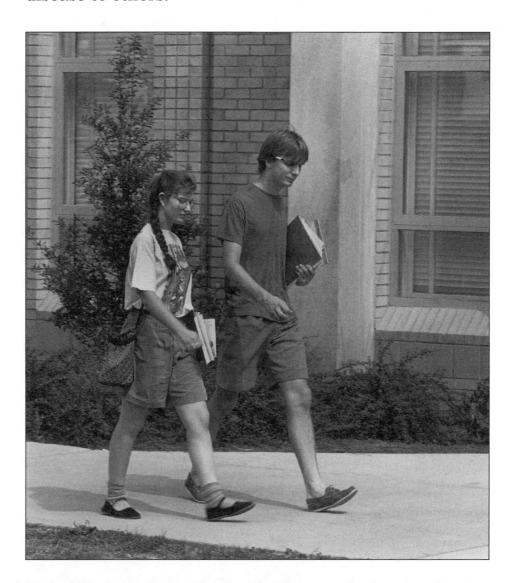

Teens who date can protect themselves from STDs by choosing abstinence.

FOUR SEXUALLY TRANSMITTED DISEASES

Disease	Pathogen	Symptoms	Treatment
chlamydia	bacteria	Symptoms can appear 5 to 12 days after infection. At times there are no symptoms. Sometimes there is discharge from the sex organs. If a person with the disease is not treated, the person may not be able to reproduce.	antibiotics
genital herpes	virus	Symptoms can appear 2 to 12 days after infection. Symptoms include painful blisters, burning, and redness of sex organs. Sometimes there are no symptoms. Pregnant females can infect their unborn babies during birth.	no cure
gonorrhea	bacteria	Symptoms can appear 2 to 9 days after infection. Females often have no symptoms. Males may feel pain when they urinate. Males may have discharge from their sex organ. Pregnant females can infect their unborn babies during birth. The disease can cause a person to be unable to reproduce.	antibiotics
syphilis	bacteria	Syphilis has four stages if it is not treated. •*Stage 1*. Symptoms appear about 3 weeks after infection. A painless sore appears on the sex organs. The sore disappears in about 3 weeks. •*Stage 2*. Symptoms begin 6 weeks to 6 months later. The person has rash and fever for several weeks. The rash and fever will disappear without treatment. •*Stage 3*. There are no symptoms for 5 to 20 years. •*Stage 4*. Bacteria attack the body organs. The disease can cause blindness, brain damage, or heart disease. A person with syphilis can die at this stage. Babies of pregnant females who have syphilis may be born dead, or they may die shortly after birth.	Antibiotics can cure syphilis during stages 1, 2, and 3.

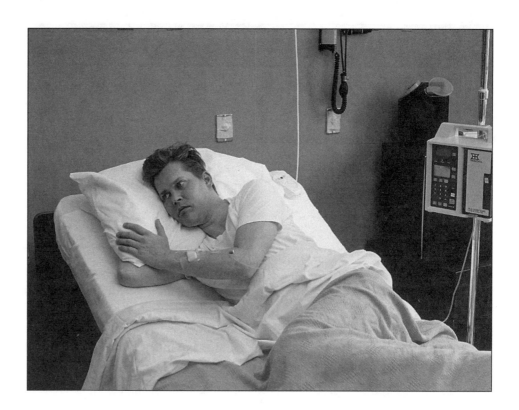

People who are sick with AIDS are very sick. Their immune systems cannot fight germs.

What Is AIDS?

AIDS stands for acquired immune deficiency syndrome. AIDS is always caused by the **HIV virus**. Once the virus enters your body, you are infected for the rest of your life. There is no cure at this time for AIDS. Most people who get sick with AIDS will die.

The HIV virus lives in blood and fluids from the sex organs. The HIV virus kills special white blood cells called T-helper cells. Your immune system cannot fight other diseases without these T-helper cells. People who are sick with AIDS die because their immune systems cannot fight germs and disease.

There is a big difference between having the HIV virus in your body and being sick with AIDS. People who are sick with AIDS are very ill. But most people who get AIDS have the HIV virus in their bodies for 8 to 11 years before they become sick. During this time people who have the HIV virus may look and feel fine. Most people do not even know they have the HIV virus. But they can spread the virus to many people. Most people who have the HIV virus will one day get sick with AIDS and later die.

The Three Stages of AIDS

There are three stages of the AIDS disease. During the first stage, the HIV virus enters the body. This stage can last as long as 11 years. People may feel fine. But the virus is slowly destroying the body's T-helper cells. The immune system becomes weak.

During stage two people may still feel fine most of the time. But they will get more infections. One of these diseases is a kind of pneumonia. People also lose weight during this stage.

During stage three the immune system no longer works. People who are sick with AIDS often have fever. They feel very tired and weak. They no longer look well because they have lost far too much weight. Many people who are sick with AIDS get a skin cancer that causes ugly purple marks. Some people who are sick with AIDS lose their hair. They may get skin sores. Many people who are sick with AIDS will die in about two years.

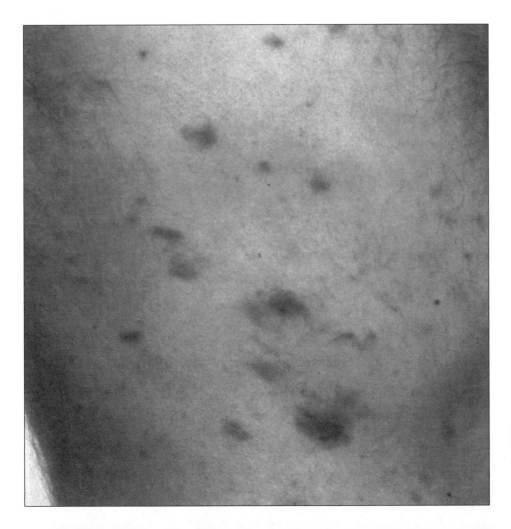

Many people with AIDS get this kind of skin cancer. It causes ugly purple marks.

Getting AIDS and Testing for AIDS

Most people get AIDS through intimate sexual behavior with an infected person. About one fourth of the people with the HIV virus are drug abusers. They get AIDS by sharing drug needles with an infected person. Pregnant females with the HIV virus can pass the HIV virus to their babies. About one third of these babies will get AIDS and later die. Teen-agers who use these risk behaviors can get AIDS.

The chart on this page lists risk behaviors that can cause you to get AIDS. It also lists safe behaviors that never spread AIDS.

If you use any of the risk behaviors, you should have an AIDS blood test. You can learn if you have the HIV virus. You should go for a blood test three months after you think you were infected. People who think or know they have the virus should not spread it to others.

You can find out from your school nurse or doctor where to get an AIDS test and counseling. Health clinics also have this information. Testing is **confidential** or **anonymous**. You can also learn about testing and counseling by calling the AIDS hot line in your town or city. You can also call 1-800-342-AIDS.

Confidential means secret.

Anonymous means someone whose name is not known.

How AIDS Is Spread

Risk Behaviors:

1. You can get AIDS by having intimate sexual behavior with a person who has the HIV virus.
2. You can get AIDS by sharing drug needles with an infected person.
3. Pregnant females with the HIV virus pass the disease to their unborn babies.

Safe Behaviors:

1. You cannot get AIDS by touching, hugging, kissing, or shaking hands with a person with AIDS.
2. You cannot get AIDS by sharing cups, towels, and other objects that were used by a person with AIDS.
3. You cannot get AIDS from animal or insect bites.
4. You cannot get AIDS by using the same bathroom that is used by a person with AIDS.
5. You cannot get AIDS from giving blood to a blood bank.

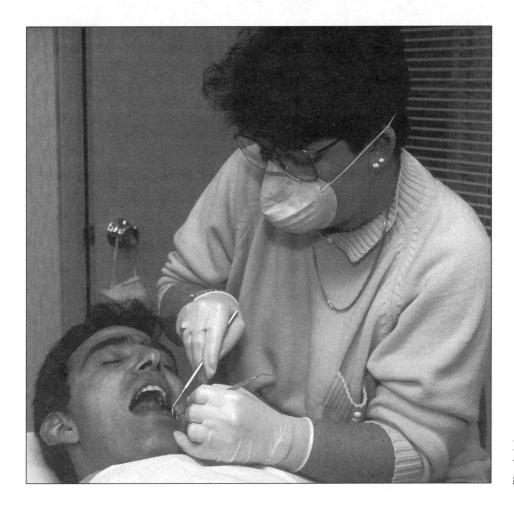

Dentists and health care workers should wear latex gloves when they treat you.

Protecting Yourself from AIDS

These rules will prevent you from getting AIDS.
1. Do not have intimate sexual behavior.
2. Say no to drugs.
3. Do not share needles that are used to **pierce** ears or make tattoos.
4. Always wear latex gloves if you must touch other people's blood.
5. Ask your dentist and other health care workers to wear latex gloves when treating you.

Pierce means to make a hole in something. Many people pierce their ears and wear earrings in the holes.

Refusal skills can help you say no to intimate sexual behavior. You can say, "I am not ready for intimate sexual behavior." Or you might say, "I believe in waiting until I am married to have intimate sexual behavior." Always say no to risk behaviors that can spread AIDS.

Protect yourself from AIDS and STDs. This can help you have a long, healthy life.

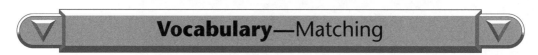

Using What You Learned

Vocabulary—Matching

Match each vocabulary word in **Group B** with a sentence from **Group A** that tells about the word. Write the letter of the correct answer on your paper.

Group A

1. This is the most common STD.

2. This comes out of an infected part of the body.

3. AIDS testing that is kept secret is called this.

4. This virus kills T-helper cells and causes AIDS.

5. A baby born to a mother with chlamydia can have this infection of the lungs.

Group B

a. discharge

b. pneumonia

c. chlamydia

d. confidential

e. HIV

Comprehension—True or False

Write **True** on your paper for each sentence that is true. Write **False** on your paper for each sentence that is false. There are two false sentences. Rewrite the false sentences to make them true.

1. The AIDS disease has only one stage.

2. You can get AIDS from having intimate sexual behavior with someone who has AIDS.

3. Pregnant females can infect their unborn babies with AIDS.

4. The HIV virus helps special white blood cells called T-helper cells.

5. Some STDs can be cured with antibiotics and other medicines.

6. Genital herpes can cause painful blisters to appear on the sex organs.

Write a sentence on your paper to answer each question.

1. How can you avoid STDs?

2. Where in the body does the HIV virus live?

3. How do most people get AIDS?

4. Why do people who are sick with AIDS die?

5. What is the first stage of the AIDS disease?

6. How can people find out if they have the HIV virus?

Critical Thinking—Drawing Conclusions

Read the paragraph. Then use the six steps to decide what to do about AIDS. Write complete sentences on your paper to answer each question.

> You have a friend who has AIDS. You enjoy spending time with this friend. But your other friends do not want you to be around this friend. They are afraid that you will get AIDS, too. Your friends start to spend less time with you.

Step 1. What is the problem?

Step 2. What are two ways to solve the problem?

Step 3. What is one consequence for each choice listed in Step 2?

Step 4. Which choice do you think is best?

Step 5. What can you do to put your decision into action?

Step 6. Think about your decision. Why was this the best choice for you?

Chapter 35

Other Diseases

Think About as You Read

- **What are the signs of a heart attack?**
- **What happens during an asthma attack?**
- **What health habits help prevent disease?**

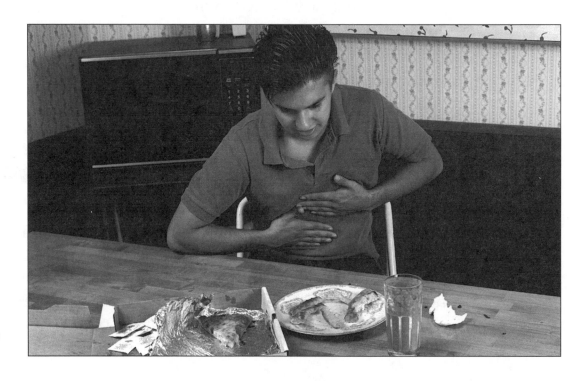

This teen has a food allergy to pizza. He became sick when he ate the pizza.

Kevin and his friends bought a pizza for lunch. Kevin knew he should not eat pizza because he has an allergy to milk. He decided to eat the pizza anyway. A short time later, Kevin got pains in his stomach.

An allergy is a **noncommunicable disease**. A noncommunicable disease does not spread from one person to another. Pathogens do not cause noncommunicable diseases. Problems inside the body cause noncommunicable diseases. In this chapter you will learn about some noncommunicable diseases.

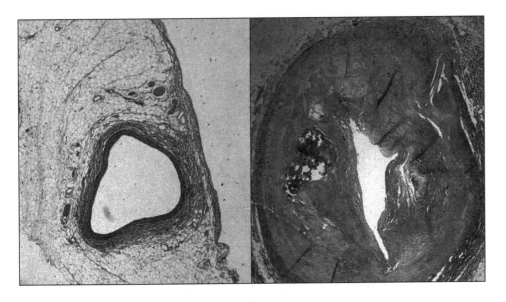

The left artery is healthy. The right artery is blocked with cholesterol.

Cardiovascular Diseases

High blood pressure and **atherosclerosis** are diseases that affect the heart and arteries. These diseases can also lead to two very dangerous cardiovascular diseases, heart attack and **stroke**.

High blood pressure can be caused by many factors. Smoking, stress, and being overweight can greatly increase your blood pressure. Eating foods that are high in fat and salt is another cause of high blood pressure. It is important to have your blood pressure checked regularly. Your doctor can help you find ways to lower your blood pressure if it is too high.

Atherosclerosis is a buildup of cholesterol and fats on the inside walls of arteries. Over many years this buildup can cause arteries to become very narrow. The heart must pump much harder to send blood through these arteries. A person with atherosclerosis is at high risk for having a heart attack or a stroke.

A heart attack can happen if an artery becomes so narrow that blood stops flowing to part of the heart. The cells in that part of the heart die. A symptom of a heart attack may be pains in the chest, arms, neck, shoulders, or jaw. Dizzy feelings, sweating, difficulty in breathing, and a sick feeling in the stomach are other possible symptoms. A person with any of these symptoms should be taken to a hospital right away.

A **stroke** is a cardiovascular disease that damages the brain. It can occur if an artery in the brain bursts or becomes blocked.

267

A stroke is a brain attack. It can occur if an artery in the brain bursts or becomes blocked. Nerve cells in part of the brain die because they cannot get oxygen. After a stroke a person may not be able to walk or talk.

Follow these five rules to help lower your risk of getting cardiovascular diseases.

1. Avoid smoking. Smoking greatly increases your risk of getting cardiovascular diseases.

2. Maintain your ideal weight. Being overweight causes your heart to work much harder.

3. Exercise regularly. Exercise makes your heart stronger and helps to lower your blood pressure.

4. Eat foods that are low in salt, fat, and cholesterol.

5. Avoid stress. Stress can increase your blood pressure and cause you to use risk behaviors.

Allergies and Asthma

More than 35 million Americans have allergies. Certain **allergens** cause allergies. The allergens may be foods, animals, plants, dust, or chemicals. Some allergies cause a person to have red eyes, a stuffy nose, or other health problems.

Allergens are any things to which people have allergies.

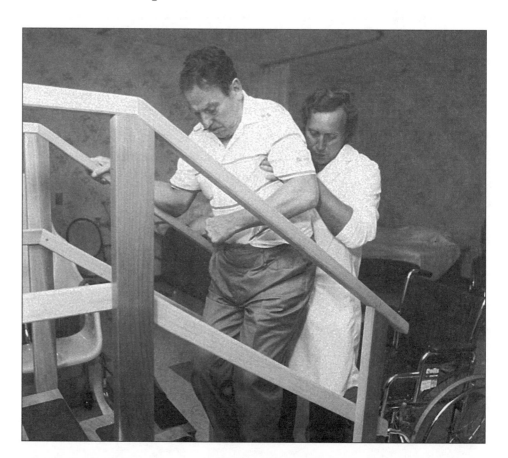

Some people cannot walk after a stroke. Medical care can help them learn to walk again.

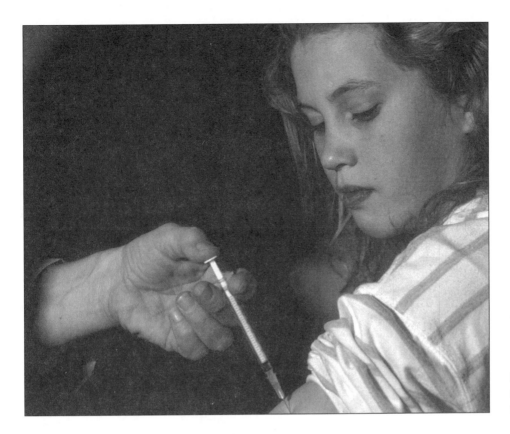

Shots can treat some allergies. The shots reduce the symptoms of allergies.

A doctor can treat allergies. Allergies cannot be cured. Your doctor can help you learn which allergens, if any, are a problem for you. Try to avoid those allergens. If you have an allergy to milk, as Kevin did, avoid all foods with milk. Your doctor can give you medicine for allergies to help you feel more comfortable. Shots can treat some allergies. The shots will reduce the symptoms of allergies.

Asthma is a lung disease. Asthma bothers millions of people. There are tiny tubes in your lungs that carry air to the air sacs. During an asthma attack, the tubes in the lungs become tight and narrow. Air cannot easily move in and out of these tight, narrow tubes. A person with asthma has a hard time breathing. The person coughs a lot during an attack. Allergies or infections cause most asthma attacks.

There is no cure for asthma. Sometimes people's asthma becomes less of a problem when a doctor treats their allergies. Different kinds of medicines can control asthma. All people with asthma need to be under the care of a doctor.

Diabetes

Diabetes is another noncommunicable disease. The body of a person with diabetes cannot use sugar in normal ways. The hormone **insulin** helps the body digest sugar. In some people with diabetes, the body does not make enough insulin. In other people who have diabetes, the body cannot use insulin to digest sugar.

Diabetes has two main symptoms. People often feel very thirsty. They also need to urinate often.

Diabetes can be controlled. People with diabetes can live a long life. They can control diabetes by exercising and eating a special diet. They may need to lose weight. Some people who have diabetes must take insulin shots. Sometimes people take pills to control diabetes.

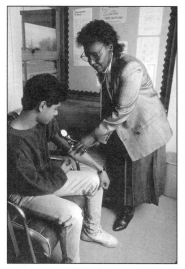

Have your blood pressure checked at least once a year.

Protecting Yourself from Disease

Choose healthy behaviors that protect your health. These eight rules can help you prevent many diseases.

1. Do not smoke.
2. Exercise at least three times a week.
3. Eat a diet that is high in fiber. Your diet should be low in fat, sugar, salt, and cholesterol. Avoid red meat, egg yolks, and fried foods.
4. Have your blood pressure checked at least once each year.
5. Get enough sleep.
6. Learn how to live with stress. Talk about your feelings with people you trust. Stress weakens your immune system. Stress also makes your blood vessels become narrower.
7. Wash your hands often with soap and warm water.
8. Take a bath or shower every day.

Healthy behaviors help you live with less disease. Choose healthy behaviors to reach your goal of wellness.

Using What You Learned

Vocabulary—Find the Meaning

Write on your paper the word or words that best complete each sentence.

1. A _____ disease cannot be spread from one person to another.

   communicable   **noncommunicable**   **sexually transmitted**

2. The hormone _____ helps the body digest sugar.

   insulin   **fiber**   **cholesterol**

3. Atherosclerosis can cause a _____ or a heart attack.

   pathogen   **chemical**   **stroke**

4. People with _____ cannot use sugar in normal ways.

   diabetes   **atherosclerosis**   **allergies**

5. A build-up of _____ narrows the inside of your arteries.

   asthma   **insulin**   **cholesterol**

Comprehension—Write the Questions

Below are the answers for some questions from this chapter. Read each answer. Then write on your paper a possible question to go with each answer. Use the question words to help you.

1. What _____ ?

   Cholesterol is a fatty substance that can build up inside arteries.

2. How _____ ?

   A person can help lower his or her blood pressure by exercising.

3. When _____ ?

   A person can have a stroke when an artery in the brain is blocked.

4. What _____ ?

   Allergies and infections cause most asthma attacks.

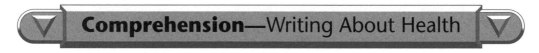

Comprehension—Writing About Health

Answer the following question in complete sentences on your paper.

What are four healthy behaviors that help prevent many diseases?

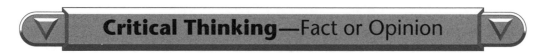

Critical Thinking—Fact or Opinion

Write **Fact** on your paper for each fact below. Write **Opinion** for each opinion. You should find six sentences that are opinions.

1. People with diabetes often feel thirsty and need to urinate.
2. Finding a friend with whom you can talk is the hardest part of learning to live with stress.
3. The most painful part of having a heart attack is the chest pains.
4. The tubes in the lungs become tight and narrow when a person has an asthma attack.
5. It is easy to protect yourself from diseases.
6. Pathogens do not cause noncommunicable diseases.
7. It is easier to live with allergies than any other noncommunicable disease.
8. Smoking and stress can lead to high blood pressure.
9. Stress weakens your immune system and makes your blood vessels narrow.
10. Chest pains are one sign that a person might be having a heart attack.
11. Getting enough sleep is the best way to avoid diseases.
12. A stroke is the worst kind of cardiovascular disease.

Cancer

Think About as You Read

- **What are the seven signs of cancer?**
- **How do doctors treat cancer?**
- **How can you avoid getting cancer?**

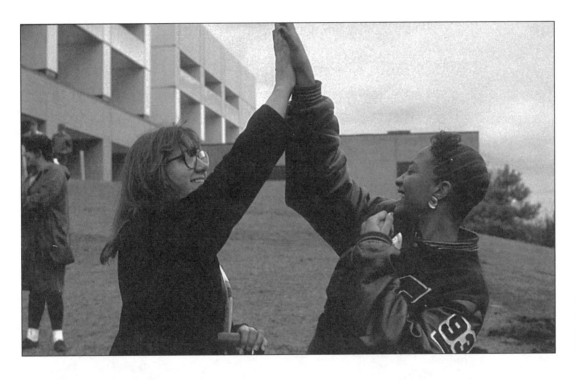

This person had cancer. She was treated and cured. She is healthy today.

Gina is 15 years old. She knows she is lucky because she is healthy today. Six years ago Gina had a type of cancer called **leukemia**. Gina has had many treatments. Now she is cured. In this chapter you will learn how to treat and prevent cancer.

Understanding Cancer

Cancer cells reproduce faster than normal cells. Cancer cells damage your body's healthy cells and organs.

Leukemia causes the body to make too many white blood cells that are not normal. These white blood cells cannot fight germs.

A **tumor** is a lump that grows in the body. A tumor can be made of normal cells or cancer cells.

Cancer cells often grow into a **tumor**. A tumor can grow in any part of the body. Cancer cells can break away from the tumor. The blood carries cancer cells to other parts of the body. The cancer cells form new tumors in different parts of the body. A person becomes very sick when cancer spreads throughout the body.

Most lumps in the body are not cancer. You should always have your doctor check all lumps.

Doctors can cure some cancer. They must find and treat small tumors before the tumors grow and spread throughout the body.

Three Types of Cancer

There are many types of cancer. All cancers are noncommunicable diseases. Skin cancer, lung cancer, and leukemia are three common types of cancer.

Spending too much time in the sun for many years causes skin cancers. Always use a sunscreen lotion when you are in the sun. The lotion should have an SPF number of 15 or higher. When you are in the sun, wear a hat and lightweight clothes to protect yourself. Doctors can cure most skin cancers that are found early.

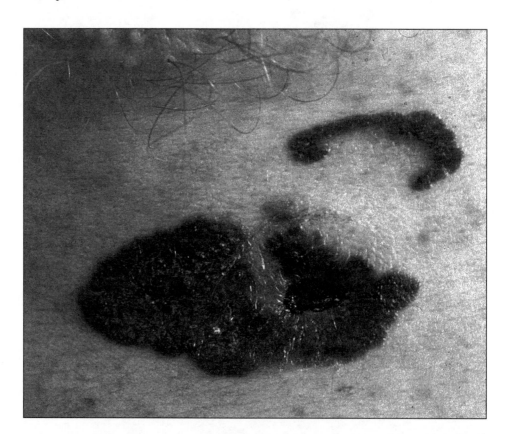

Spending too much time in the sun can cause skin cancers. How can you protect your skin?

274

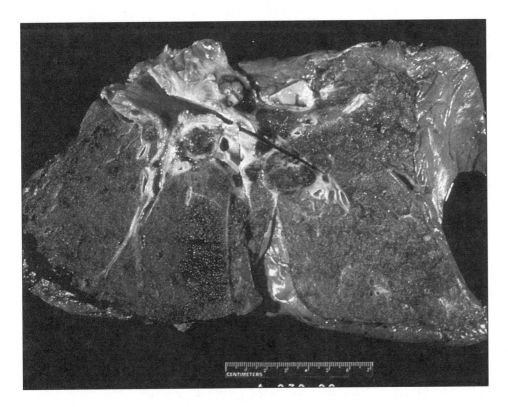

This lung belonged to a smoker. The lung cancer was caused by cigarette smoking.

Lung cancer kills more Americans than any other cancer. Smoking causes most cases of lung cancer. Lung cancer is very hard to cure.

Leukemia is the most common cancer in children. Adults also get this disease. There are many ways to treat this cancer. Most children can be cured of leukemia.

Seven Warning Signs of Cancer

The American Cancer Society tells people to look for the seven signs of cancer. See your doctor if you have any of these warning signs for more than two weeks.

1. A sore on any part of the body does not heal.
2. A small or large lump is in the breast or any part of the body.
3. A mole or wart changes in size, shape, or color.
4. You have a cough or a hoarse voice.
5. There is a change in your **bowel** or bladder habits.
6. You have difficulty swallowing or a sick feeling in the stomach because your body cannot digest food.
7. You have unusual bleeding or discharge.

The intestine is also called the **bowel**. Food passes from the stomach into your bowels. Solid waste leaves your body when you have a bowel movement.

Finding, Treating, and Preventing Cancer

Males between the ages of 15 and 34 sometimes get cancer in their testes. Males should check their testes once a month. They should see a doctor if they think there are changes in their testes.

Females can get cancer in their breasts. The disease can be cured by removing the tumor. Females should check their breasts for lumps once a month. The best time to do this is soon after menstruation has stopped.

Some females get cancer in their reproductive organs. A **Pap test** can find this type of cancer. Females should have a Pap test once a year.

Doctors start a person's cancer treatment soon after the cancer is found. Surgery removes tumors made of cancer cells that are in small areas of the body. **Radiation** kills cancer cells in the body. **Chemotherapy** kills cancer cells that might have spread throughout the body. People are cured when they have no sign of cancer for five years.

Here are six ways to avoid getting cancer.

1. Do not smoke or use tobacco.
2. Do not breathe dangerous chemicals.
3. Eat foods that are high in fiber and low in fat.
4. Eat many kinds of fruits and vegetables.
5. Do not drink alcohol.
6. Wear a sunscreen lotion in the sun.

You can protect yourself against cancer. Having good health habits will help you.

Radiation is a treatment for cancer. Very strong rays are aimed at cancer cells to kill them.

Chemotherapy is the treatment of cancer with powerful medicines.

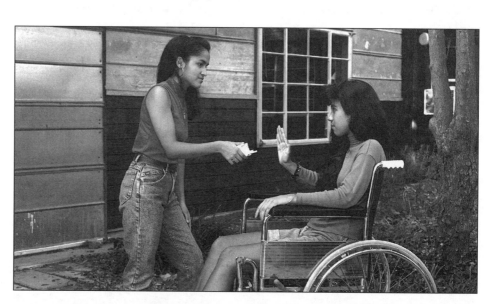

Say no to cigarettes. You will help protect yourself from lung cancer.

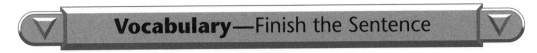

Using What You Learned

Choose a word or words from the box to complete each sentence. Write the correct answers on your paper.

bowel	tumor	Pap test
surgery	chemotherapy	leukemia

1. A _____ is a lump in the body made of normal cells or cancer cells.

2. A cancer called _____ causes the body to make too many white blood cells that cannot fight germs.

3. Tumors that are made of cancer cells can be removed from small areas of the body using _____ .

4. A _____ can be used to find cancer in a female's reproductive organs.

5. Radiation and _____ kill cancer cells in the body.

6. One warning sign of cancer might be a change in your _____ or bladder habits.

Comprehension—Write the Answer

Write a sentence on your paper to answer each question.

1. What happens when cancer cells break away from a tumor?

2. Why shouldn't you spend too much time in the sun?

3. What is the most common cancer in children?

4. What should you do if you think you have cancer?

5. Where do males sometimes get cancer?

Comprehension—True or False

Write **True** on your paper for each sentence that is true. Write **False** on your paper for each sentence that is false. There are three false sentences. Rewrite the false sentences on your paper to make them true.

1. Cancer cells reproduce more slowly than normal cells.

2. Most lumps in the body are not cancer.

3. All cancers are noncommunicable diseases.

4. Smoking causes most cases of leukemia.

5. Females sometimes get cancer in their reproductive organs.

6. Chemotherapy is the treatment of cancer with powerful medicines.

7. Lung cancer is very easy to cure.

Critical Thinking—Categories

Read the words in each group. Decide how they are alike. Find the best title in the box for each group. Write the title on your paper.

| Cancer Treatments | Types of Cancer |
| Ways to Prevent Cancer | Signs of Cancer |

1. skin cancer
   lung cancer
   leukemia

2. sore that won't heal
   change in a mole or wart
   small or large lump

3. surgery
   radiation
   chemotherapy

4. wear a sunscreen lotion
   eat foods that are high in fiber
      and low in fat
   don't smoke or use tobacco

278

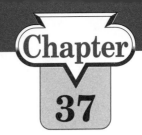

Understanding and Treating Disease

Think About as You Read

- What can doctors learn from blood tests and urine tests?
- How does a doctor make a diagnosis?
- What new ways of doing surgery help people?

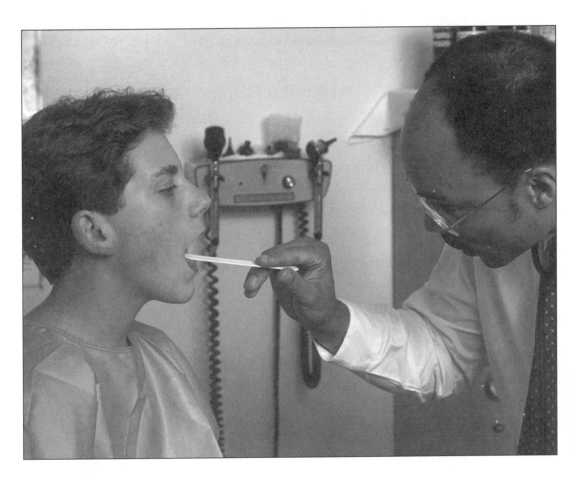

A doctor will use different tests to learn what is causing this patient's sore throat.

Each year scientists invent new medicines to treat disease. Doctors must know why a person is sick to order the correct medicine. Better ways of making a **diagnosis** help doctors learn why people are sick. In this chapter you will learn about the diagnosis and treatment of disease.

A **diagnosis** is the name given to a disease or health condition. A doctor makes a diagnosis after examining and studying the symptoms of a patient.

279

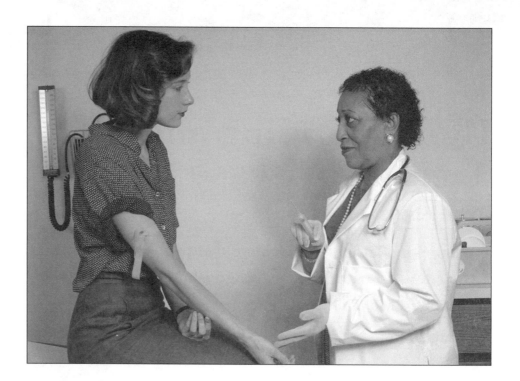

Blood tests show the health of the blood. These tests can show many diseases and allergies.

Many Ways of Making a Diagnosis

Doctors use blood tests and urine tests to make a diagnosis. Blood tests show the health of the blood. These tests show many allergies and diseases. They also show other problems. Urine tests show if a person has an infection. Sugar in the urine is a sign of diabetes. Blood in the urine is a sign of infection or disease.

Doctors use a special machine to record a person's heartbeat. The machine records on a sheet of paper the pattern of the heartbeat. This record is a **cardiogram**. Sometimes the pattern on the cardiogram is not normal. This is a sign of heart disease.

Doctors use x-rays to get information about bones and teeth. A **mammogram** helps doctors find breast cancer. This x-ray can show very tiny cancer tumors. Doctors can remove small tumors before they grow and spread.

Ultrasound is the use of sound waves to outline the shape of a person's body parts.

Ultrasound helps doctors learn what is happening inside the body. Doctors use ultrasound to learn about the health of the body's organs. Ultrasound helps doctors find tumors. It helps doctors learn about the health of an unborn baby.

280

Treatments Using Medicine

Today doctors use many different antibiotics to cure diseases. Scientists are always making new antibiotics. They are also working on new drugs to cure cancer.

Years ago doctors gave all medicines in pills, liquids, or shots. Now some people wear medicine patches on their skin. The medicine slowly goes through the skin and into the blood. Medicine patches help many people who have heart disease.

Surgery to Treat Disease

Organ **transplants** save the lives of many people with diseased organs. Sometimes a person's heart, kidneys, or other organs are so diseased that the person will die. Doctors may use surgery to remove a diseased organ. Then they replace that organ with a healthy organ from a **donor**.

Transplants are body parts from a healthy person that replace the diseased parts of another person.

A **donor** is the person from whom body parts are taken to use in a transplant. A donor can be dead or living.

This healthy kidney will be given to a person who has a diseased kidney.

Rejection can be a problem for a person who has an organ transplant. The body's immune system attacks the organ from the donor. There are new drugs to stop rejection of transplants. These drugs are helping people with transplants live for many years.

Bypass surgery helps many people who have narrow arteries. Their arteries are blocked with cholesterol. Doctors can do bypass surgery on a person to prevent a heart attack. During surgery doctors remove a short piece of a blood vessel from the chest or leg of the person. Doctors then attach that piece to the blocked artery. The blood flows more easily through the new blood vessels. The heart gets the blood it needs. Then it does not have to work as hard.

Sometimes diseases or accidents destroy parts of the body. Doctors now replace diseased joints with **artificial** ones. They can replace a diseased lens of the eye with an artificial one.

The diagnosis and treatment of disease improves every year. You can learn about the newest ways by watching the news on TV. You can also learn about them by reading the newspaper. This information can help you choose the best health care. Your decisions can help you reach the goal of wellness.

Artificial describes something that is made by people.

Some doctors do laser surgery. Strong beams of light cut and repair the body.

282

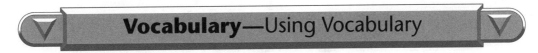

Using What You Learned

Vocabulary—Using Vocabulary

Use the word or words to write a complete sentence on your paper about understanding and treating disease.

1. transplants
2. artificial
3. cardiogram
4. ultrasound
5. bypass surgery

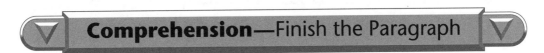

Comprehension—Finish the Paragraph

Number your paper from 1 to 6. Use a word from the box to finish each sentence. Write the correct answers on your paper.

teeth	organs	urine
diagnosis	pattern	mammogram

   Doctors make a __(1)__ by using different tests and machines. Blood tests and __(2)__ tests can tell a doctor if a person has allergies, an infection, or a disease. Doctors use a machine to see the __(3)__ of a person's heartbeat. They take x-rays to check a person's __(4)__ and bones. A __(5)__ helps doctors find breast cancer. Doctors use ultrasound to find out about the health of the body's __(6)__ .

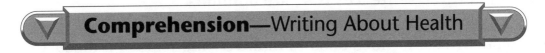

Comprehension—Writing About Health

Answer the following question in complete sentences on your paper.

What happens during bypass surgery?

283

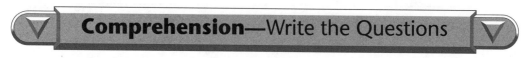

Comprehension—Write the Questions

Below are the answers for some questions from this chapter. Read each answer. Then write on your paper a possible question to go with each answer. Use the question words to help you.

1. When _____ ?

   A doctor makes a diagnosis after examining and studying a patient's symptoms.

2. Why _____ ?

   Doctors use blood tests and urine tests to make a diagnosis.

3. What _____ ?

   Sugar in the urine is a sign of diabetes.

4. How _____ ?

   You can learn about the newest ways of treating disease by watching the news on TV.

5. What _____ ?

   A transplant is a body part taken from a healthy donor to replace a diseased part of another person.

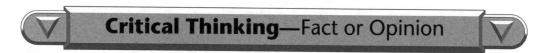

Critical Thinking—Fact or Opinion

Write **Fact** on your paper for each fact below. Write **Opinion** for each opinion. You should find three sentences that are opinions.

1. Blood tests are sometimes used to make a diagnosis of a disease.

2. A mammogram can help doctors find breast cancer.

3. Bypass surgery is the best way to prevent a heart attack.

4. Rejection can be a problem for a person who has an organ transplant.

5. Artificial joints are used to replace diseased joints.

6. It is better to use a medicine patch than medicine in a pill, liquid, or shot.

7. Reading a newspaper is the fastest way to learn about new treatments for disease.

8. A donor for a transplant can be dead or living.

9. A cardiogram can show whether a person's heartbeat pattern is normal.

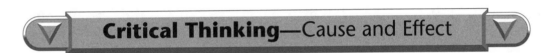

Critical Thinking—Cause and Effect

Write sentences on your paper by matching each cause on the left with an effect on the right.

Cause

1. Many people suffer from disease, so _____

2. Your doctor thinks you have a bladder infection, so _____

3. A person's immune system attacks an organ from a donor, so _____

4. The doctor wants to check the health of a pregnant female's unborn baby, so _____

5. A person's arteries are blocked with cholesterol, so _____

6. Disease has destroyed a joint in the body, so _____

Effect

a. the doctor uses ultrasound on the pregnant female.

b. your doctor gives you a urine test.

c. scientists invent new medicines.

d. the joint is replaced with an artificial one.

e. the person is given drugs to prevent rejection of the organ.

f. a person may have bypass surgery.

Chart A: How Many Calories Do Your Activities Burn?

Activity	Calories Burned in an Hour	Benefits
sleeping	65	body rests, relaxes, and repairs itself
sitting	80	no physical fitness benefits
watching TV	80	no physical fitness benefits
bowling	240	relaxing, no physical fitness benefits
baseball	300	little benefit to heart, builds muscles in arms
floor exercises	330	little benefit to heart, builds strong muscles, increases flexibility
fast walking	400	very good for heart, builds muscles in legs
fast bicycle riding	480	very good for heart, builds strong muscles
ice skating, roller skating	420	very good for heart and lungs, builds strong muscles in arms and legs
fast swimming	500	very good for heart and lungs, builds strong muscles, increases flexibility
jogging	500	very good for heart, builds leg muscles
handball	660	very good for heart, builds muscles, increases flexibility
football	600	very good for heart, builds muscles, increases flexibility
running	660	very good for heart, builds leg muscles
basketball	600	very good for heart, builds muscles, increases flexibility
jumping rope	700	very good for heart, builds arm and leg muscles

Chart B: Calories and Fats in Foods

Type of Food	Food	Calories	Fat (grams in a serving)
Meat, fish, or chicken	1 small hamburger with bread	250	10
	1 small fried chicken breast (with skin)	364	19
	1 small roasted chicken breast (with skin)	193	8
	1 small roasted chicken breast (without skin)	142	3
	1 slice of bologna	89	8
	2 ounces of canned tuna in water	60	1
	2 ounces of canned tuna in oil	150	10
Milk and cheese	1 cup of skim milk	90	less than 1 gram
	1 cup of whole milk	157	9
	1 ounce of American cheese	105	9
Snacks	1 ounce of potato chips	160	10
	1 ounce of pretzels	110	1
	2 cups of plain popcorn	60	less than 1 gram
	1 ounce of tortilla chips	140	6
	1 chocolate candy bar	240	14
	1 cup of ice cream	270	14
	1 cup of frozen nonfat yogurt	150	0
Fruits and vegetables	1 apple	80	0
	1 orange	62	0
	1 plain garden salad	70	0
	$\frac{1}{2}$ cup of cooked broccoli	25	0
	1 corn on the cob	120	1
	1 baked potato	220	0
	1 large serving of French fries	285	14
Baked foods	2 slices of white bread	140	2
	1 large bagel	230	1
	1 chocolate-covered donut	205	9
	2 small chocolate chip cookies	130	5
	1 slice of chocolate cake with icing	378	11

Chart C: First Aid

Injury	Symptoms	First Aid Treatment
Shock	very fast pulse; blood pressure drops; victim may feel weak, thirsty, and/or confused	1. Call EMS. 2. Help victim lie on his/her back with legs slightly raised. 3. Cover victim with a blanket.
Fainting	victim falls to ground and becomes unconscious	1. Leave victim lying down. 2. Raise victim's legs slightly. 3. Check breathing of victim. Start rescue breathing if breathing has stopped. 4. Call EMS if victim does not wake up in a few minutes. 5. Get medical help when victim wakes up.
Breathing stops	no air comes out of nose or mouth, chest stops moving, lips and fingernails turn blue, victim becomes unconscious, no pulse	1. Call EMS. 2. Do rescue breathing until breathing starts again or EMS arrives.
Heart attack	pain in chest; possible pain in arms, neck, and/or jaw; difficulty breathing; shortness of breath; dizzy; sweating; lips and skin may turn blue; indigestion; victim might become unconscious	1. Call EMS at once. 2. Person trained in CPR can begin doing CPR if heart stops beating. 3. Call victim's doctor if there is time. 4. Keep victim warm and comfortable. 5. Start rescue breathing if victim stops breathing.
Nosebleed	blood flows from nose	1. Have victim sit up and lean forward. 2. Press both nostrils of victim together. Have victim breathe through mouth for 10–15 minutes. 3. Call a doctor if bleeding does not stop after 10–15 minutes.
Heat stroke	skin is very red and hot, no sweating, body temperature rises fast, victim feels weak, pulse is fast and weak, victim may feel faint or become unconscious	1. Undress victim. 2. Place victim in the shade or a cool place if possible. 3. Place victim in a tub of cool water or wrap a cold, wet towel around victim. 4. Call EMS.
Broken bone	pain and swelling around the injury; victim cannot use the injured hand, leg, arm, or foot	1. Call EMS. 2. Treat for shock. 3. Avoid moving person until help arrives. 4. If victim must be moved, place injured arm or leg in a splint. Splint in the position found. Tie splint to arm or leg at points above and below the injury.
Eye injury	pain and redness in eye	1. Wash victim's eye with clean water for 10–20 minutes. Pour water from inner corner of eye toward outer corner. 2. Cover eye with sterile pad. 3. Have victim see eye doctor.

Chart D: Home Safety

Problem	How to Be Safe
Being home alone	1. Never open the front door for a person without first checking to find out who wants to come in. Do not open the door to strangers. 2. Never allow strangers to come into your home. 3. Call 911 or the operator if there is an emergency. 4. When you get telephone calls, do not tell people that you are home alone. Instead tell them your parents are not able to come to the phone.
Poisons	1. Buy medicines and cleansers in childproof containers. 2. Check expiration dates on all medicines. Flush old medicine down the toilet. Check with your pharmacist if you have questions. 3. Keep all poisons, chemicals, and medicines in places children cannot reach. 4. Keep chemicals, cleansers, and medicines in the containers they were packed. 5. Call the poison control center or EMS before you try to help someone who has swallowed a poison.
Food poisoning	1. Never eat food from rusted, leaking, or swollen cans. 2. Check expiration dates on food. Do not eat food that is older than the expiration date. 3. Wash tops of cans before opening them. 4. Do not eat raw meat, chicken, fish, or eggs.
Kitchen accidents	1. Do not leave small children alone in the kitchen. 2. Never allow children to play with plastic bags. 3. Do not wear long, loose sleeves when cooking. They can catch on fire. 4. Keep rags, paper, and towels away from the stove. 5. Keep a fire extinguisher in the kitchen to put out fires. Know how to use it to put out fires.
Accidents in the bathroom	1. Use plastic cups and bottles. 2. Wipe all spills from the floor. 3. Never leave small children alone in the bathroom. Never leave small children alone in the bathtub. 4. Do not leave medicine in a medicine chest that small children can reach or open. 5. Never use electrical appliances in or near water.
Storage areas	1. Do not keep old clothes, newspapers, and furniture that people no longer use. 2. Keep storage areas locked so children cannot go into them. 3. Keep flammable liquids in their containers. Keep flammable liquids away from heat or fire.

Chart E: Drugs Used in Substance Abuse

Drug Group	Drug	What do people call it?	Can people buy the drug legally?	How do people get the drug into their bodies?
Stimulants	cocaine	coke, snow	no	sniff it, inject it, smoke it
	crack	rock	no	smoke it
	amphetamines	speed, uppers, pep pills	yes, with a prescription	swallow pills, inject it
Hemp Plant	marijuana	pot, grass, dope	no	smoke it, eat it
Depressants	barbiturates	downers	yes, with a prescription	swallow pills
	tranquilizers	Valium, Librium	yes, with a prescription	swallow pills
	alcohol	booze	yes, if you have reached the legal age of your state	swallow it

What happens right after a person uses the drug?	What effects might the drug have on a person who uses the drug for a long time?	What happens during withdrawal?
The person feels very high, then feels very sad; has a loss of appetite; has nervous feelings; has a fast heartbeat; has high blood pressure; or cannot sleep.	The person may have strong emotional dependence on the drug, develop tolerance for larger amounts of the drug, feel very sad when the drug wears off, have violent behavior, suffer heart attacks, or die.	The person may feel a very strong hunger for the drug or feel very tired and sad.
The person feels alert and full of energy, cannot sleep, experiences fast breathing and fast heartbeat, has a loss of appetite, or dies.	The person may have emotional dependence on the drug, have tolerance for larger amounts of the drug, have poor nutrition, have violent behavior, or suffer brain damage.	The person may feel very tired and sad.
The person feels high, cannot think or remember clearly, or has red eyes.	The person may have emotional dependence on the drug, have tolerance for larger amounts of the drug, suffer damage to the lungs, or have lung cancer.	unknown
The person feels sleepy, calm, and relaxed; has slow heartbeat and slow breathing; has stomachache; has poor memory; makes poor decisions; has poor speech; or feels dizzy.	The person may have emotional and physical dependence on the drug, feel very tired or sad, suffer damage to the body's systems, or overdose and die.	The person may be nervous, have body shakes, be unable to sleep, or die.

Chart E : Drugs Used in Substance Abuse

Drug Group	Drug	What do people call it?	Can people buy the drug legally?	How do people get the drug into their bodies?
Narcotics	heroin	junk, horse	no	inject it, inhale it, smoke it
	methadone	Dolophine	yes, with a prescription	swallow it, inject it
	codeine	codeine in cough medicine or Tylenol with codeine	yes, with a prescription	swallow it
Inhalants	airplane glue gasoline shellac nail polish remover		Yes; inhalants are found in common household products.	inhale it
Hallucinogens	PCP	angel dust	no	swallow it, smoke it, inhale it, inject it
	LSD	acid	no	swallow it
	mescaline	mesc	no	swallow it, sometimes smoke it
Steroids	Anatrol Winstrol		yes, with a prescription	swallow it, inject it

292

What happens right after a person uses the drug?	What effects might the drug have on a person who uses the drug for a long time?	What happens during withdrawal?
The person feels no pain, feels sleepy, has happy and calm feelings, or has stomachache.	The person may have strong emotional and physical dependence on the drug, have tolerance for larger doses of the drug, or overdose and die.	The person may have fever, body shakes, sweating, chills, or vomiting. The person may die.
The person has poor body movements, has a cough, feels tired, is confused, or has slow heartbeat and slow breathing. At times the person may be unconscious.	The person may have emotional dependence on the drug; have violent behavior; suffer damage to the liver, brain, and blood cells; have tolerance for larger doses of the drug; or die.	unknown
The person imagines seeing and hearing beautiful or scary sights and sounds, has loss of appetite, or is nervous.	The person may have emotional dependence on the drug, have violent behavior, suffer lung damage or brain damage, have emotional problems, or have flashbacks.	unknown
The person builds body muscles quickly, gains weight quickly, or has acne.	The person may have violent behavior, feel very sad, and may suffer damage to the heart and the liver.	unknown

abdomen page 110
The abdomen is the part of your body that is below your chest and above your hips.

abdominal thrust page 110
The abdominal thrust can be used to save a person who is choking.

abstinence page 188
Abstinence is choosing not to do something. People may choose not to have intimate sexual behavior.

abuse page 91
Abuse takes place when one person hurts another in a way that is not an accident.

acceptance page 14
Acceptance is the feeling that others like you and enjoy being with you.

acids page 53
Acids are chemicals with a sour taste. Acids in vomit can damage the teeth and throat.

acne page 65
A person has acne when tiny openings in the skin become blocked with oil.

addicts page 227
Addicts are people with such strong dependence on drugs that they cannot stop using them.

adrenal glands page 173
Your adrenal glands make a hormone that helps the body handle fear and danger.

adrenaline page 28
Adrenaline is made by the body and helps prepare the body for stress.

ads page 123
Ads tell what is special or good about a product or service.

aerobic page 60
An aerobic exercise helps the heart become stronger.

affection page 14
Affection is the love that you give or get from others.

agencies page 133
Agencies are government offices that do certain kinds of work.

AIDS page 188
AIDS is a disease in which the body cannot fight germs. AIDS can be spread through body fluids. There is no cure for AIDS.

air sacs page 162
Air sacs are tiny bags of air in the lungs. Air sacs are surrounded by blood vessels.

alcoholics page 237
Alcoholics are people who have the disease of alcoholism.

Alcoholics Anonymous page 238
Alcoholics Anonymous is a group of recovering alcoholics who help each other avoid alcohol.

alcoholism page 237
Alcoholism is a disease in which a person's need to drink alcohol is strong. The person cannot control the need to drink.

allergens page 268
Allergens are any things to which people have allergies.

allergies page 138
Allergies cause a person to have a runny or stuffy nose, have breathing problems, or have other health problems. Allergies are caused by certain foods, plants, or other things that don't bother many other people.

amino acids page 38
Amino acids are substances that make up proteins. They help the body to grow and repair itself.

anonymous page 262
Anonymous means someone whose name is not known.

anorexia nervosa page 53
Anorexia nervosa is an eating disorder. People with anorexia nervosa eat only very small amounts of food to avoid gaining weight. They sometimes starve to death because they do not get enough calories and nutrients.

antibiotics page 78
Medicines called antibiotics are used to fight diseases caused by bacteria.

antibodies page 252
Antibodies are made by white blood cells to destroy pathogens.

arteries page 59
Your arteries are tubes that carry blood from your heart to different body parts.

arthritis page 131
Arthritis is a disease that causes pain and stiffness in the body's joints.

artificial page 282
Artificial describes something that is made by people.

asbestos page 164
Asbestos is used to make a building material that does not burn. Asbestos was used in the ceilings or walls of older buildings.

asthma page 269
Asthma is a lung disease. A person who has asthma has a hard time breathing air in and out of the lungs.

astigmatism page 77
An astigmatism is an eye problem that causes objects to look blurred.

atherosclerosis page 267
Atherosclerosis is a disease in which cholesterol builds up on the inside walls of the arteries.

attract page 116
To attract means to draw an object or person to oneself.

bacteria page 64
Bacteria are very tiny living things that can sometimes cause you to become sick.

balanced diet page 44
A balanced diet means eating enough servings from each of the food groups. A balanced diet provides the right amount of calories and nutrients.

binge page 53
Binge eating is when someone eats huge amounts of food at one time.

bladder page 165
Your bladder is the organ that holds urine until it leaves the body.

blood pressure page 44
Blood pressure is the force of the blood as it moves against the walls of the body's blood vessels.

blood vessels page 155
Blood vessels are the different kinds of tubes that carry blood throughout the body.

bowel page 275
The intestine is also called the bowel. Food passes from the stomach into your bowels. Solid waste leaves your body when you have a bowel movement.

braces page 73
The wires and bands that are used to move and straighten teeth are braces.

broiled page 43
Broiled food is cooked over an open flame or under the flame in the broiler of an oven.

budget   page 123
A budget is a plan for spending money.

bulimia   page 53
Bulimia is an eating disorder. People who have it do binge eating. People with bulimia do not get enough nutrients.

bypass surgery   page 282
Bypass surgery is used to make new blood vessels for carrying blood to the heart. The new blood vessels are made from blood vessels in the legs or chest.

calories   page 37
The energy in food is measured in calories.

cancer   page 43
Cancer is a disease in which unhealthy cells multiply too rapidly and destroy healthy body parts.

capillaries   page 155
Capillaries are very tiny blood vessels that connect arteries and veins. Capillaries carry blood, oxygen, and nutrients to the body cells.

carbohydrates   page 37
Carbohydrates are nutrients that give the body energy.

carbon dioxide   page 156
When cells use nutrients and oxygen, they make a gas called carbon dioxide. Carbon dioxide leaves the body when you breathe out.

cardiogram   page 280
A cardiogram is a record on paper of the pattern of a person's heartbeat.

cardiovascular system   page 59
Your cardiovascular system includes your heart, blood vessels, and blood. This system brings oxygen and nutrients to all parts of your body.

cerebellum   page 171
Your cerebellum is the part of the brain that controls the way your body moves.

cerebrum   page 170
Your cerebrum is the part of the brain that controls thinking, talking, and learning.

Cesarean section   page 200
A Cesarean section is an operation that might be done if a mother is having trouble delivering her baby.

chemotherapy   page 276
Chemotherapy is the treatment of cancer with powerful medicines.

child abusers   page 208
Child abusers are people who hurt children in ways that are not accidents.

chlamydia   page 258
Chlamydia is an STD that is caused by bacteria.

cholesterol   page 40
Cholesterol is a fatty substance that is made by the body and is also found in certain foods. Too much cholesterol in the blood can cause heart disease.

circulatory system   page 155
Your circulatory system is the group of body parts that sends blood through your body.

clinics   page 138
Clinics are places where doctors and nurses treat health problems.

cocaine   page 227
Cocaine is an illegal drug that speeds up the nervous system. Its effects last a short time.

codeine   page 226
Codeine is a prescription drug that reduces pain.

doses   page 226
Doses are amounts of medicine that a person takes at one time.

drug abuse   page 219
Drug abuse is using a drug in a way that is not correct. Drug abuse is also using a drug for no medical reason.

eating disorders   page 52
People with eating disorders are afraid of gaining weight. Eating disorders cause very unhealthy eating habits that harm the body.

emotional health   page 5
Emotional health is the way you live with your feelings. Good emotional health means that you have good feelings about yourself.

emotions   page 12
Emotions are strong feelings, such as love, joy, anger, hate, or fear.

enamel   page 70
Your teeth have a hard, white covering called enamel.

endocrine system   page 172
Your endocrine system makes chemicals that help your body work and grow properly.

endurance   page 60
You have endurance when you can do activities, like running, for a long period of time.

energy   page 28
Energy is the strength to work or do other things.

environment   page 202
The environment includes the people, places, and objects that are around a person.

enzymes   page 154
Enzymes are chemicals made by the body and used to break down food.

Eustachian tube   page 78
The Eustachian tube connects the ear, nose, and throat.

evacuate   page 116
To evacuate means to leave.

expiration date   page 218
The expiration date is the last date that you should use a medicine.

extended family   page 179
An extended family has one or both parents, one or more children, and other family members living in a home.

fad   page 124
A fad is a style that lasts for a short time.

Fallopian tubes   page 194
The egg cell travels through one of the Fallopian tubes as it leaves an ovary.

farsighted   page 76
People are farsighted when things that are far away look clear, but things that are close look blurred.

fertilized egg   page 198
A fertilized egg is an egg that has joined with a sperm and can grow into a baby.

fiber   page 38
Fiber is a carbohydrate from plants that helps the body remove wastes but is not digested. The fiber in a food has no calories.

fibers   page 170
Thin, threadlike parts attached to nerve cells are nerve fibers.

fight or flight response   page 28
The fight or flight response protects the body from stress and danger. During this response the body releases adrenaline to give you extra energy.

first-degree burn page 108

A first-degree burn is the least dangerous burn. It makes the skin painful and red.

flammable page 100

Things that can easily catch on fire are flammable.

flexibility page 60

Your flexibility allows you to stretch your body in many directions.

floss page 72

You floss when you clean between your teeth, using a strong waxed or unwaxed thread called dental floss.

fluoride page 72

A chemical that protects teeth from decay is fluoride.

food processors page 98

Food processors are electric machines that chop, grind, and blend foods.

foster family page 179

A foster family is a family where adults care for one or more children because the children's natural parents cannot take care of them.

fungus page 66

A fungus is a very tiny, nongreen plant that sometimes causes disease.

garbage disposals page 98

Garbage disposals in sinks grind food to get rid of it.

generic page 139

Generic means a product has the same purpose and ingredients as a product with a company name. A generic product usually costs less.

glands page 65

Glands are inside your body. Some glands make sweat or oil. Other glands make hormones.

glaucoma page 77

The eye disease called glaucoma is caused by too much pressure within the eye.

goggles page 78

Goggles are safety glasses that are worn to protect the eyes.

grams page 47

Grams are measures of weight.

guardian page 94

A guardian is an adult who is responsible for taking care of the needs of a young person.

hallucinogens page 228

Hallucinogens are drugs that change the way people see, hear, smell, taste, and feel.

health maintenance organization (HMO) page 140

A health maintenance organization is a group of doctors and hospitals that have agreed to provide medical services at a special rate to its members.

heroin page 217

Heroin is a dangerous, habit-forming drug.

high page 220

To feel high means to have a good feeling that lasts a short time. People sometimes get high from abusing drugs.

HIV page 260

HIV is the virus that causes AIDS.

homicide page 92

The killing of one person by another person is a homicide.

hormones page 172

Hormones are made by endocrine glands to help the body grow or stay healthy. Hormones enter the blood. The blood carries the hormones to the parts of the body where they are needed.

hospitalization page 140
Hospitalization is insurance that pays for part of the cost of being in a hospital.

ideal weight page 51
Your ideal weight is the weight that is right for someone of your age, height, and bone size.

immune system page 252
The immune system is the different kinds of white blood cells and antibodies that work together to fight disease.

immunity page 252
Immunity means the body can fight off a disease without becoming sick.

immunization page 138
An immunization is a type of medicine that stops a person from getting a disease.

infected page 65
An area of the body becomes infected when bacteria or other germs attack and grow there.

ingredients page 47
Ingredients are the parts of a food that are mixed with others when cooking, baking, or packaging.

inhalants page 229
People sniff inhalants in order to have pleasant feelings.

inherited page 202
Inherited means a person received certain traits from his or her parents.

insulin page 270
Insulin is a hormone that helps the body digest sugar.

involuntary muscles page 149
Involuntary muscles receive messages from the brain so they can work on their own to control many organs of the body.

joints page 148
Joints are places where bones meet.

kidneys page 165
The kidneys are a pair of organs that remove liquid waste from the blood.

labor page 199
Labor is the physical work done by a female's body to give birth to a baby.

large intestine page 155
The large intestine stores solid waste until the solid waste leaves the body.

latex page 107
Latex is a strong, stretchy material like rubber.

leukemia page 273
Leukemia causes the body to make too many white blood cells that are not normal. These white blood cells cannot fight germs.

life cycle page 198
The life cycle is the five stages of life from birth until death.

long-term goals page 22
Long-term goals are goals that may take you one or more years to reach.

major medical page 140
Major medical is insurance that helps pay for large medical bills. It pays for surgery and expensive health tests.

malocclusion page 73
A person has a malocclusion when the teeth in the mouth are crooked, crowded, or do not fit together well when chewing.

mammogram page 280
A mammogram is an x-ray picture of a breast.

marijuana page 226
Marijuana is an illegal drug that people use to feel high.

300

mature   page 192
Mature describes something or someone that is fully grown or fully developed.

Medicaid   page 140
Medicaid helps people who do not earn much money pay for visits to clinics, hospital stays, medicines, and certain doctor bills.

Medicare   page 140
Medicare pays for hospital stays of people who are at least 65 years old.

medulla   page 171
The medulla is the part of the brain that controls the body's systems.

menstruation   page 194
Menstruation is the three-to-seven-day period when the egg cell flows out of the uterus with some blood.

minerals   page 37
Minerals are nutrients needed by the body to provide healthy teeth, muscles, bones, and blood cells.

miracles   page 130
Miracles are things that cannot be explained.

moles   page 66
Black or brown spots on the skin are moles.

mucus   page 79
Mucus is a sticky liquid that is made by the body. Mucus helps protect the body against germs and dirt.

narcotic   page 226
A narcotic is a drug that reduces pain and causes dependence.

natural disaster   page 114
A natural disaster is an accident caused by nature.

natural parent   page 179
A natural parent is related to the child by blood.

nearsighted   page 76
People are nearsighted when close things can be seen clearly, but things that are farther away look blurred.

neglect   page 91
Young people suffer from neglect when their needs are not met by the adult who takes care of them.

nervous system   page 170
Your nervous system controls your thinking and the way your body moves and works.

nicotine   page 242
Nicotine is a drug in tobacco that causes dependence.

nitrites   page 44
Nitrites are chemicals added to certain fish and meats, such as hot dogs and sliced sandwich meats. Nitrites may be harmful to your health.

noncommunicable disease
page 266
A noncommunicable disease does not spread from one person to another. It is not caused by pathogens.

nutrients   page 37
Nutrients are substances in food that the body needs for health and life.

nutrition   page 36
Nutrition is the food needed by the body for life and growth.

opposite sex   page 187
The opposite sex is the one that is different from your own. If you are a male, a member of the opposite sex is a female.

organs page 147
Organs are made of large groups of cells. Each body organ has a certain job to do.

orthodontists page 73
Orthodontists are dentists who are trained to correct malocclusions.

osteoporosis page 59
Osteoporosis is a problem in which the bones lose calcium. As a result the bones become weaker and break easily.

outlet page 99
An outlet is a place for plugging in an electric appliance.

ovaries page 194
Ovaries are female sex glands that produce female hormones and egg cells.

oxygen page 147
Oxygen is a gas that has no color or smell.

Pap test page 276
A Pap test is a test to check for cancer in a female's reproductive organs.

passive smoker page 243
A passive smoker breathes smoke from the cigarettes, pipes, or cigars of other people.

pathogens page 251
Pathogens are very tiny living things that cause disease. They are too small to be seen without a microscope.

pedestrians page 101
People who walk down the street are pedestrians.

peer pressure page 29
Peer pressure is the control over your decisions that other people of your age try to have.

peers page 13
Your peers are people who are about the same age as you.

perspiration page 164
Perspiration is a liquid that is made by the body. It contains water, salt, and wastes from your blood.

pharmacist page 139
A pharmacist is a person who prepares medicine your doctor has ordered for you.

physical fitness page 58
You have good physical fitness when you can use your body to work, exercise, and play without getting tired quickly.

physical health page 5
Physical health is how you take care of your body. Eating healthy foods, exercising, and sleeping enough are ways to take care of your physical health.

pierce page 263
Pierce means to make a hole in something. Many people pierce their ears and wear earrings in the holes.

pituitary gland page 172
The pituitary gland makes hormones that control other endocrine glands as well as the growth of the bones.

plaque page 71
Bacteria make a sticky covering called plaque on teeth.

pneumonia page 258
Pneumonia is an infection of the lungs.

polluted page 163
Polluted describes something that is dirty and unhealthy.

pores page 65
Your pores are tiny openings in the skin. Oil and sweat come out of your pores.

posture page 59
Your posture is the way you carry your body when sitting and standing.

pregnancy page 188
Pregnancy is having one or more unborn children growing inside a female's body.

prejudices page 23
All prejudices are unfair ideas about other people.

pressure page 28
Pressure is a strong demand.

product page 123
A product is anything that is made.

proteins page 37
Proteins are nutrients that the body uses for growth and repair.

puberty page 191
Puberty is the time when the sex organs and the sex glands begin to work.

quack page 131
A quack is a person who sells useless or harmful health care products or services.

quackery page 130
Quackery is the selling of useless or harmful health care products or services that are supposed to improve health.

rabies page 108
Rabies is a disease that can kill animals and people.

radiation page 276
Radiation is a treatment for cancer. Very strong rays are aimed at cancer cells to kill them.

rape page 92
Rape is a crime where force is used by an attacker to perform sexual acts on another person.

recovering alcoholics page 238
Recovering alcoholics have learned how to stop drinking alcohol.

refusal skills page 31
Refusal skills are skills used to say no to peer pressure and to avoid risk behaviors.

rejection page 282
Rejection happens when the immune system attacks the organ a person receives during a transplant. People can die from organ rejection.

relationships page 184
Relationships are the way you get along with others.

reproduce page 251
To reproduce means to make other living things. People reproduce by having babies. Bacteria make more bacteria when they reproduce.

reproductive organs page 192
Reproductive organs are the parts of the body that allow males and females to produce children.

respiratory system page 161
Your respiratory system is a group of organs that work for the body to take in oxygen and give off carbon dioxide.

responsibilities page 180
Responsibilities are jobs you do that show you can be trusted to do things well.

risk behaviors page 5
Risk behaviors are behaviors that can harm your health. Risk behaviors stop people from reaching the goal of wellness.

scoliosis page 149
Scoliosis is an unhealthy curving of the spine.

second-degree burn page 108
A second-degree burn is a dangerous burn. The skin may be painful and have blisters.

self-esteem   page 20
Self-esteem is the good feelings you have about yourself.

sexual   page 187
Sexual describes anything that has to do with being a male or a female.

sexually transmitted diseases
page 188
Sexually transmitted diseases are diseases that can be spread from person to person through intimate sexual behavior.

short-term goals   page 22
Short-term goals are goals that you are able to reach in days or months.

shoulder harness   page 101
A shoulder harness is the part of the seat belt worn across the shoulder. It helps protect a person from being thrown forward during a car accident.

side effects   page 218
Side effects are unpleasant and sometimes dangerous effects medicines have on the body.

sidestream smoke   page 243
Sidestream smoke is the smoke sent into the air by the burning end of a cigarette, pipe, or cigar.

small intestine   page 154
The small intestine is a long tube where most of the digestion of food is finished.

smoked   page 44
Smoked foods are prepared for future use by using smoke. Bacon is a food that is sometimes smoked.

smoke detectors   page 100
Smoke detectors are small machines that buzz when there is smoke in a room or hallway.

smokeless tobacco   page 242
Smokeless tobacco is made from tobacco leaves and is chewed, dipped, or sniffed.

social health   page 5
Social health is the way you get along with others. Good social health means you try to get along with family and friends.

sperm cells   page 193
Sperm cells are male reproductive cells.

SPF   page 66
SPF stands for sun protection factor. An SPF number tells how much protection a sunscreen provides.

spinal cord   page 170
Your spinal cord is a thick row of nerves that goes down the center of your back.

starch   page 38
Starch is a carbohydrate that provides longer-lasting energy. Most of your calories should come from starches.

sterile   page 107
A sterile bandage is free from dirt or germs.

stimulants   page 227
Stimulants are drugs that speed up the body's systems.

strep bacteria   page 253
Strep bacteria cause sore throats and other diseases.

stress   page 27
Stress is the way the body responds to physical, emotional, and social demands. Every person feels stress each day.

stroke   page 267
A stroke is a disease that damages the brain. It happens when blood cannot flow through a blocked artery to the brain.

sunscreen lotion page 66
A sunscreen lotion blocks the sun's harmful rays from damaging your skin.

surgery page 138
Surgery is the use of medical tools to operate on the body.

survive page 115
To survive means to go on living even though there are problems.

symptoms page 258
Symptoms are signs of a disease.

systems page 147
Systems are groups of organs that work together to do different jobs for the body.

tartar page 71
The hard material that is caused by plaque and forms on the teeth near the gums is tartar.

testes page 193
The testes are the male endocrine glands that make male sex hormones.

tetanus page 107
Tetanus is a dangerous disease that is caused by a bacteria that enters the body through a wound.

third-degree burn page 109
A third-degree burn is the most dangerous burn. It damages every layer of the skin.

throat culture page 253
A throat culture is the growth of bacteria from the throat. The bacteria grow in a small, closed dish. A throat culture helps a doctor learn what kind of pathogen is causing a person's sore throat.

thyroid gland page 173
The thyroid gland makes a hormone that controls the speed with which the body uses food.

tolerance page 220
Tolerance means the body needs more of a drug to get the same feeling it once felt with smaller amounts.

traditional family page 179
A traditional family has a mother, a father, and one or more children.

traits page 202
Traits are characteristics, such as skin and eye color, that belong to each person.

tranquilizers page 226
Tranquilizers are prescription drugs that have a calming effect because they slow down the nervous system.

transplants page 281
Transplants are body parts from a healthy person that replace the diseased parts of another person.

tread page 102
To tread water is to keep your head above water and the rest of your body straight up and down. Do this with an up-and-down movement of your feet and sometimes your arms.

tumor page 274
A tumor is a lump that grows in the body. A tumor can be made of normal cells or cancer cells.

ultrasound page 280
Ultrasound is the use of sound waves to outline the shape of a person's body parts.

ultraviolet rays page 78
Ultraviolet rays are harmful rays from the sun.

umbilical cord page 199
The umbilical cord is a thick cord made of blood vessels that connects the baby's navel to its mother's uterus.

uncomfortable   page 92
You are uncomfortable when someone does or says things that make you feel afraid.

unconscious   page 109
People are unconscious when they have passed out, and they cannot feel things or think.

unit price   page 124
The unit price is the price of one ounce, pound, quart, or other measurement of a product.

urinary system   page 161
Your urinary system is a group of organs that remove liquid waste from the body.

urinate   page 165
To urinate is to rid the body of urine.

urine   page 165
Urine is the liquid waste that is made by the kidneys.

uterus   page 194
The uterus is the female organ where a developing baby grows during pregnancy.

vaccines   page 252
Vaccines are medicines that help the body make antibodies. Vaccines protect you from getting certain diseases.

vagina   page 199
The vagina is the part of a female's body that goes from the uterus to outside the body.

values   page 180
Your values are your ideas about what is important.

veins   page 155
Veins are blood vessels that carry blood from other parts of the body back to the heart.

victims   page 92
Victims are people who are harmed or killed by another person.

violent   page 92
To be violent means to act with strong force.

virus   page 250
A virus is a very tiny living thing that causes disease. A virus can multiply and grow only when it is inside the body's cells.

vitamins   page 37
Vitamins are a group of nutrients that the body must have in small amounts in order to work and grow as it should.

voluntary muscles   page 148
You can control voluntary muscles in order to move your body.

vomit   page 53
To vomit is to throw up food from the stomach.

wellness   page 5
Wellness means having good physical, social, and emotional health. The highest health goal is wellness.

withdrawal   page 227
Withdrawal is the body's reaction to not having a drug on which it is dependent.

workout   page 61
A workout is a group of exercises that help make the heart and other muscles stronger.

wounds   page 107
Wounds are cuts or scratches or bites.

yogurt   page 46
Yogurt is a thick, soft food made from milk.

oxygen, 147, 153, 156, 161–162, 164, 169

P

Pap test, 276
parenthood, 210–211
passive smoker, 243–244
pathogens, 251, 252, 266
PCP, 228, 292–293
pedestrian safety, 101
peer pressure, 29–31, 124, 207, 221, 230, 244
peers, 13
personal exercise program, 60–61
personal health
  ear care, 78–79
  eye care, 76–78
  and grooming, 84–85
  hair care, 67, 83, 84
  nail care, 67, 83, 84
  physical fitness, 58–61, 82–84
  planning for, 82–85
  records, 137–139
  skin care, 64–66, 83, 84
  for teeth, 70–73
perspiration, 164
pharmacist, 139
phone numbers for emergencies, 106
physical abuse, 91–92
physical dependence, 219, 227, 236, 290–293
physical fitness, 58–61, 82–84
physical health, 5, 13, 51, 59, 173, 211, 236
pimples, 65
pituitary gland, 172, 193
plaque, 71, 72
pneumonia, 254, 258, 261
poisoning, 109
polluted air, 163
pool safety, 101–102

pores, 65
posture, 59, 84, 149, 150
pregnancy
  alcohol use during, 236
  beginning of, 193, 198–199
  care during, 200
  HIV and, 262
  intimate sexual behavior as cause of, 188
  length of, 199, 201
  marriage and, 207
  sexually transmitted diseases and, 258
  of teen-agers, 208
  tobacco use during, 200, 242
prejudices, 23
prescription drugs, 217–218, 226
pressure, 28
products, 123–126, 132, 133
proteins, 37–38, 39
puberty, 191–195, 201

Q

quack, 131
quackery, 130–133

R

rabies, 108
radiation, 276
rape, 92–93
recovering alcoholics, 238
red blood cells, 157
refusal skills, 31, 230–231, 237, 238, 245, 263
relationships, 184–188
reproduce, 251
reproductive organs, 192
rescue breathing, 111
respiratory system, 161–164
responsibilities, 180–184

restaurants, and healthy meals, 46
risk behaviors, 5–6, 15–16, 29, 188

S

safety
  from abuse, 92
  during natural disasters, 114–117
  at home, 97–100
  need for, 14–15
  outside the home, 101–102
  preparing for emergencies, 114–115
  protecting yourself, 90–94
scoliosis, 149
second-degree burn, 108
self-esteem, 20–24, 51, 53, 59, 84, 91, 92, 93, 180, 187, 195, 221, 235, 244, 245
sex glands, 193
sexual, 187
sexual abuse, 91
sexual behavior, 187–188, 195, 208, 262
sexually transmitted diseases, 188, 257–259, 263
shock, 106
shoes, 126
short-term goals, 22
shoulder harness, 101
side effects, 218
sidestream smoke, 243–244
skin cancer, 66, 274
skin care, 64–66, 83
sleep, 83, 85
small intestine, 154, 171
smoke detectors, 100
smoked foods, 44

Acknowledgments, continued

Unit 7 pp.144–145 © Tony Freeman/PhotoEdit; p.146 © Tony Freeman/PhotoEdit; p.147 © R. Becker/Custom Medical Stock Photo; p.149 © Tony Freeman/PhotoEdit; p.150 © Jeffry Myers/Stock Boston; p.153 © Robert Brenner/PhotoEdit; p.157 © J. Berndt/Stock Boston; p.158 © Myrleen Ferguson/PhotoEdit; p.164 © Spencer Grant/Photo Researchers; p.166 © Michael Newman/PhotoEdit; p.169 © Myrleen Ferguson/PhotoEdit; p.172 © Tony Freeman/PhotoEdit. Unit 8 pp.176–177 © Myrleen Ferguson/PhotoEdit; p.178 © Tony Freeman/PhotoEdit; p.179 © Robert Brenner/PhotoEdit; p.180 © Tony Freeman/PhotoEdit; p.181 © Lawrence Migdale/Photo Researchers; p.184 © Spencer Grant/Stock Boston; p.185 © Elizabeth Crews/Stock Boston; p.186 © Peter Menzel/Stock Boston; p.187 © Mary Kate Denny/PhotoEdit; p.191 © Bill Bachman/Photo Researchers; p.192 © Tony Freeman/PhotoEdit; p.193 © Barbara Rios/Photo Researchers; p.194 © Barbara Rios/Photo Researchers; p.195 © Tony Freeman/PhotoEdit; p.198 (egg) © Richard Rawlins/Custom Medical Stock Photo, (sperm) © J.L. Carson/Custom Medical Stock Photo; p.200 © Billy Barnes/Stock Boston; p.201 © Nancy Durrell McKenna/Photo Researchers; p.202 © Jeffry Myers/Stock Boston; p.203 © Myrleen Ferguson/PhotoEdit; p.206 © Robert Brenner/PhotoEdit; p.207 © Ulrike Welsch/PhotoEdit; p.208 © Gale Zucker/Stock Boston; p.209 © Myrleen Ferguson/PhotoEdit; p.210 © Kathy Sloane/Photo Researchers; p.211 © Tony Freeman/PhotoEdit. Unit 9 pp.214–215 © Tony Freeman/PhotoEdit; p.216 © Focus On Sports; p.217 © Tony Freeman/PhotoEdit; p.218 © Siu Biomed Comm/Custom Medical Stock Photo; p.219 © Charles Gatewood/Stock Boston; p.220 © Tom Prettyman/PhotoEdit; p.221 © Michael Weisbrot/Stock Boston; p.222 © Tony Freeman/PhotoEdit; p.225 © D.Cantwell/Custom Medical Stock Photo; p.226 © Frank Siteman/Stock Boston; p.227 © Charles Gatewood/Stock Boston; p.228 © Tony Freeman/PhotoEdit; p.229 © Elizabeth Zuckerman/PhotoEdit; p.230 © L. Druskis/Stock Boston; p.231 © Bob Daemmrich/Stock Boston; p.234 © Mary Kate Denny/PhotoEdit; p.235 © Tony Freeman/PhotoEdit; p.236 © Robert Brenner/PhotoEdit; p.237 © Mary Kate Denny/PhotoEdit; p.238 © Jeffrey Myers/Stock Boston; p.241 © Charles Gatewood/Stock Boston; p.242 © Custom Medical Stock Photo; p.243 © Custom Medical Stock Photo; p.244 © Elizabeth Zuckerman/PhotoEdit. Unit 10 pp.248–249 © Biomedical Communications/Photo Researchers; p.250 © Bernard Peirre Wolff/Photo Researchers; p.251 © Mary Kate Denny/PhotoEdit; p.252 © Custom Medical Stock Photo; p.253 © L. Druskis/Stock Boston; p.257 Center For Disease Control; p.258 ©Tim Barnwell/Stock Boston; p.260 © Thomas Bowman/PhotoEdit; p.261 © National Medical Slide/Custom Medical Stock Photo; p.263 © Robert Brenner/PhotoEdit; p.267 (healthy) © Custom Medical Stock Photo, (diseased) ©Roseman/Custom Medical Stock Photo; p.268 © Custom Medical Stock Photo; p.269 © Scott Camazine/Photo Researchers; p.270 © Bob Daemmrich/Stock Boston; p.273 © Steve Skjold/PhotoEdit; p.274 © Custom Medical Stock Photo; p.275 © Custom Medical Stock Photo; p.279 © Blair Seitz/Photo Researchers; p.280 © L. Steinmark/Custom Medical Stock Photo; p.281 © Custom Medical Stock Photo; p.282 © Custom Medical Stock Photo.